Serving People with
Food Allergies

Serving People with Food Allergies

Kitchen Management and Menu Creation

Joel J. Schaefer

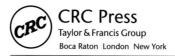

CRC Press
Taylor & Francis Group
Boca Raton London New York

CRC Press is an imprint of the
Taylor & Francis Group, an **informa** business

CRC Press
Taylor & Francis Group
6000 Broken Sound Parkway NW, Suite 300
Boca Raton, FL 33487-2742

© 2011 by Taylor and Francis Group, LLC
CRC Press is an imprint of Taylor & Francis Group, an Informa business

No claim to original U.S. Government works

Printed and bound in India by Replika Press Pvt. Ltd.
10 9 8 7 6 5 4 3 2 1

International Standard Book Number: 978-1-4398-2804-5 (Hardback)

Visit the Taylor & Francis Web site at
http://www.taylorandfrancis.com

and the CRC Press Web site at
http://www.crcpress.com

CONTENTS

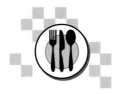

PART I   KNOWLEDGE

PART II   SKILLS

Chapter 5   Getting Started   **105**

Chapter 6   Service Management   **127**

I dedicate this book to the people who suffer from food allergies and special diets that want to enjoy a safely prepared meal with their family and friends in restaurants.

FOREWORD

In this book, Joel Schaefer, former Culinary Development and Special Dietary Needs Manager at Walt Disney World® Resort, shares his vast knowledge about how to serve guests with food allergies and other special diets. Joel developed the Special Diet Request program for Walt Disney World® Resort and helped thousands of families enjoy a dream trip to Disney World in Orlando, Florida.

In fact, that's where I met Joel. I was there to present a seminar on gluten-free cooking to his staff and I was greatly impressed with their system that assures each guest has a safe culinary experience. Understandably, his program received many glowing praises from happy families across the nation.

Now, Joel shares his vast expertise with the rest of the food service industry, helping them to understand what food allergies are, how to train workers to meet the special requests of diners, and providing recipes for dishes that meet those requests. He focuses on the eight major food culprits—wheat, milk, eggs, soy, peanuts, tree nuts, fish, and shellfish—but also offers help for other special diets such as autism and diabetes.

Back when Joel and I were initially struggling with our respective food culprits (Joel's dairy; mine wheat) there were only 6 million Americans with food allergies. Today, the Food & Anaphylaxis Network says there are 12 million. The incidence of food or digestive allergies among children is particularly alarming, growing 18% between 1997 and 2007, according to the Centers for Disease Control.

Celiac disease, an autoimmune form of intolerance to gluten (a protein in wheat) but not an allergy, has also increased. In the 1990s, we thought celiac disease occurred in 1 in 300 people. Thanks to Dr. Alessio Fasano's research, we know that it is closer to 1 in 100 (3 million Americans). Recent research by Dr. Joseph Murray at the Mayo Clinic shows that it is nearly 5 times more common than it was 50 years ago and he calls it "a public health issue." In addition, Fasano estimates that about 6 or 7 times more people have non-celiac gluten intolerance, which equates to another 20 million who can't eat wheat.

Given the increases in food allergies and celiac disease, along with the 1.5 million autistic children and the 18 million diagnosed diabetics, one thing is certain: given these huge numbers, many of these people are likely to show up in your food service institution hoping you can feed them. Eating should be a natural and enjoyable activity, but there is no magic pill to cure any food sensitivity. The only treatment is to avoid the offending foods, replacing them with safe ingredients, and that's why Joel's book is a must-have resource for the food service industry.

I am honored to know Joel and greatly appreciate all he has done for the millions of us who have to choose our foods carefully. On behalf of all of us, thank you, Joel!

Carol Fenster, PhD
President/Founder, Savory Palate, Inc., author of 100 Best Gluten-Free Recipes

INTRODUCTION:
THE UNPLEASANT PAST
LEADS TO A BRIGHT FUTURE

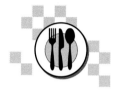

CHILDHOOD

As a child, I had problems with my digestive system. I experienced bouts of constipation and diarrhea, and had a rough time gaining weight. When I was five years old I was hospitalized for tests because of night terrors. The doctors thought there was a link between the night terrors and my digestive system. They tested me for a variety of food allergies, milk being one of them, but could not find any connection. Luckily, I grew out of my night terrors but still had problems with my digestive system.

ADOLESCENCE

In my teen years, I became very familiar with allergy pills. After my breakfast of cereal and milk, almost immediately I would start sneezing and having problems breathing. My nose would get plugged up and my eyes would start to itch. My mom said it was probably "morning allergies" since there was substantial pollen and dust in the air from all of the fruit and nut orchards in the area. That made sense, but I wanted to be sure, so I went to an allergist for testing. I was pricked, prodded, and drained of blood but the results were only the basics: dust, mites, oak, and so forth. I was not tested for food allergies, since the doctors did not think it was relevant.

At the age of 16, I entered the food service industry as a dishwasher at a local coffee shop. Matters only got worst. Since I was exposed to "all-you-can-eat" breakfast, lunch, and dinner (I worked every shift possible to support my bowling habit), my digestive problems started to go to my head, literally. I started to get severe migraines. They were so bad that everything hurt from my eyes, ears, and face to my hair. There would be times that other employees would find me sitting in the freezer with my hands cradling my face because the extreme cold would help numb the pain.

ADULTHOOD

From the age of 18 to 23, I worked in a variety of kitchens as a cook and kitchen manager. I continued to take allergy pills and frequented the freezer, praying that the pain would go away. At the age of 23, I was 6 foot, 4 inches tall, and weighed 135 pounds. Can you imagine me in a chef's outfit with a tall toque? I looked like a walking Q-tip.

At 23, I had been in the food service industry for 7 years and was really good at cooking but wanted to learn more, so I decided to go to culinary school.

In 1988, I had the opportunity to attend the California Culinary Academy in San Francisco. Now the real food challenge would begin since I was going to be exposed to all types of cuisines with great food and I had to try everything. Wow! Not a bad deal for someone that loved to eat. Imagine this dish: seared foie gras with grand marnier sauce, oranges, and heavy cream. It was awesome, but it did not take long for me to reach for an allergy pill and end up in the bathroom three hours later.

FINALLY FINDING THE ANSWER

For many years, I had been going to a chiropractor. Since my move to San Francisco, I had to search for a new doctor. I found one that used to be a medical physician but changed practices because he wanted to help people naturally and did not want to treat them with medications.

After a few treatments this chiropractor asked me about my diet and how I felt after eating. I told him that my diet consisted of cereal with milk, cheese sandwiches, ice cream floats, pizza, and more cheese. I went through the scenario of the allergy pills, migraine headaches, and the repeated bathroom breaks. He thought it would be a good idea for me to have a series of blood tests and the results were astounding. Cholesterol, calcium, phosphorus, and potassium were off the charts. Based on the results and my history of health issues, he put me on an elimination diet.

He started me out with eliminating all milk products. I said, "What are you saying? No cheese or ice cream? You have got to be crazy!" My chiropractor said if I wanted to feel better I had to follow this diet. So I went home and reluctantly threw out all of the milk products in my refrigerator and freezer. That did not leave me very much food, but it was worth it. Within a few weeks, I was not taking as many allergy pills, my migraines were almost gone, and I started to feel like a normal person again.

After a few weeks, I thought I was cured so I started eating cheese and ice cream again, and the symptoms came back threefold. When I went back to my chiropractor, he asked me how I was feeling. When I told him that I started eating milk products again and explained how I felt, he just shook his head. He said, "I told you if you want to feel better, you have to stay away from anything with milk, but it is your choice." "How long will I have to eat like this?" I asked. "Forever. At this time, there is no cure for food allergies. You are just going to have to live with it," he answered. That was not what I wanted to hear, but it was reality. At that time there was not a lot of material on food allergies or intolerances, or any additional advice that my chiropractor could provide. I still continued to experience minor digestive problems because of occasional cheating and not reading food labels. But all in all I was feeling much better.

PROFESSIONAL LIFE

As my professional career continued, I cannot recall encountering anyone with food allergies or food intolerances, so I felt alone. From 1994 to 1998 while I was a culinary instructor at Kapiolani Community College in Hawaii, there was not any information in textbooks about food allergies. In 1998 I had the opportunity to move to Orlando, Florida, and work at Walt Disney World Resort were I started to hear more about special diets and food allergies.

My first experience serving a person with a food allergy was in a banquet environment. The guest was an adult female with a severe allergy to peanuts. I knew very little about food allergies. I only knew that people could die from eating the wrong food, so I went to the guest's table to personally talk to her.

She was sitting alone in the back of the room, away from the buffet stations when I arrived. I talked to her and she explained that she would not eat from the buffet in fear of cross-contamination (this will be referred to as cross-contact throughout the book) and wanted to know if any of the menu items contained peanuts. She also wanted to know if we had any peanuts in our kitchen. I explained that there were no peanuts in any of the menu items but that we did have open containers of mixed nuts that included peanuts and peanut butter in the kitchen. She seemed a little nervous and asked me if I could make anything safe for her to eat. I asked her what she usually ate and we agreed on a menu of fresh fruit, baked chicken breast, and sauté vegetables. I told her it would be about 20 to 30 minutes to prepare because I had to make everything from scratch. She agreed to wait.

I was a little nervous about making her food because she seemed a little uneasy. By the time I prepared her meal and delivered it, she was gone. When I asked one of the servers where she went, he informed me that she did not feel comfortable eating here and went back to her room to eat the food she had brought with her. This was a little unsettling to me, since I had spent all that time making her a special meal and she left. Did I do something wrong? How bad could an allergy be to peanuts? This incident encouraged me to learn more about food allergies.

I did some research and found out that food allergies were not as rare as I had thought. At that time, 6 million Americans were allergic to eight common foods: milk, eggs, peanuts, tree nuts, fish, shellfish, soy, and wheat. These foods account for 90% of food allergy reactions and many more people had food intolerances or sensitivities. This was astounding! Even though I had issues with milk, I could not believe that there were so many people with food allergies. My studies in food allergy, food intolerance, and nutrition had begun.

In 2004, I became the Culinary Development and Special Dietary Needs Manager at Walt Disney World Resorts. I had the opportunity to develop the Special Dietary Request program. Over the next several years, I learned many valuable lessons and developed processes that have benefited many chefs, managers, and guests with food allergies.

In the following chapters, we will discuss the basics of food allergy and special diets. I will share my knowledge, skills, and abilities in the areas of communication, training your service and culinary teams on safe service and food preparation techniques. We will discuss how to set up your kitchen for success and provide ways to modify your menus to meet the request for meals that eliminate many of the top eight food allergens.

Since you may not have dealt with many food allergy requests in the past, you may not feel that this book is important to your food service career. Before you make that decision, think about these numbers. In the last seven years the number of Americans with a food allergy has risen from 6 million to over 12 million. This shows a definite increase in the number of food-allergic people and the numbers will continue to rise. One day, if it hasn't already happened, a customer with a food allergy will be coming to your restaurant.

AUTHOR

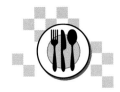

Joel J. Schaefer, CCC, CHT, is a certified Chef de Cuisine with the American Culinary Federation and a Certified Hospitality Trainer with the American Hotel and Lodging Association. Schaefer is the president of his own company, Allergy Chefs, Inc., specializing in food allergy and special diets training and product development. He has developed a unique training program called T.E.A.C.H. Food Allergen Safety for the food service industry.

Along with running his own business, Schaefer is the Research & Development Chef for AllergyFree Foods and consulting chef for the Café at Virginia College. His past experience includes manager of Product Development and Special Diets for Walt Disney World Resort; culinary nutrition instructor at Valencia Community College in Orlando, Florida; and chef instructor at Kapiolani Community College in Honolulu, Hawaii.

Over the past several years, Schaefer has been a guest speaker, an emcee, and a culinary demonstrator for various events and organizations such as the Gluten-Free Culinary Summit, the American Culinary Federation, the National Restaurant Association, the Oldways and Whole Grains Council, and the Food Allergy & Anaphylaxis Network.

Schaefer has experience in culinary education and training, product development, food allergies, special diets, and culinary demonstrating. In 2009, he was the recipient of the Michael Ty Endowment Fund, an American Culinary Federation national award, recognizing him for his educational work with children and the food service industry in the areas of nutrition and food allergy awareness.

In his free time he works with his wife, Mary, developing recipes that meet the dietary requirements for people with celiac disease, food allergies, and other health-related issues.

ACKNOWLEDGMENTS

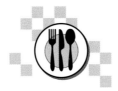

I want to thank the following individuals and organizations for their support and contributions to this manuscript: Gina Clowes, President of AllergyMoms.com; Kim Koeller, President, AllergyFree Passport® and GlutenFree Passport®; Shelley Case, BSc, RD, author of *Gluten-Free Diet: A Comprehensive Resource Guide*; Professor Jonathan Brostoff and Linda Gamlin, authors of *The Complete Guide to Food Allergy and Intolerance*; Kevin Hannaway, son of Dr. Paul J. Hannaway, MD, author of *On the Nature of Food Allergy*; The Food Allergy & Anaphylaxis Network; and Living Without® magazine.

A special thank you to my close friend Carol Fenster, PhD, author, guest speaker, and president of Savory Palate, Inc., who reviewed this manuscript and provided me with essential feedback that benefited its content. I also want to thank my friend Michael Cairns, owner of Wet Orange Studios, Orlando, Florida, for the food photography; the students of Culinard, the Culinary Institute of Virginia College in Jacksonville for helping in the preparation of the food; and the Movsovitz Group, Produce Distribution Center of Jacksonville, Florida, for supplying the produce.

I completed this manuscript with the help of my Lord, Jesus Christ and my loving wife, Mary. Mary's help in reviewing this manuscript, testing the recipes, and her continuing encouragement made this work a reality.

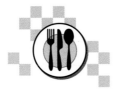

PART I

Knowledge

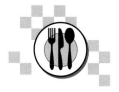

CHAPTER 1

Food Allergies and the Food Service Industry

If you are reading this book, you are one of the many food service professionals who wants to learn more about food allergies. You may be wondering why there are more customers coming into your establishment requesting meals without certain ingredients and you might be thinking, "Growing up I did not know anyone with a food allergy. How could someone be allergic to food? Why is this happening all of a sudden? What can I do to learn more about food allergies that will help me better serve these customers?"

Could taking just one bite of peanut butter kill you? The answer is yes if you are one of the 3.3 million Americans who have a food allergy to the protein found in peanuts. According to the Food Allergy & Anaphylaxis Network (FAAN), peanuts are one of the top eight foods that account for 90% of all known food allergies along with eggs, milk, fish, shellfish, soy, tree nuts, and wheat (see Figure 1.1).

Food allergies are a growing public health and safety concern in the United States and around the world. It is now becoming a major concern for governments, doctors, families, and the food service industry. As the number of food allergies increase, we need to take steps to educate ourselves and make an effort to help the families that are affected.

**Food Allergen
Wheel**

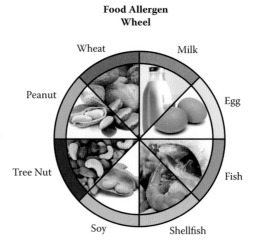

FIGURE 1.1
FOOD ALLERGEN WHEEL.

Since guests with food allergies and special diets are dining out more often, it is time to address food service concerns about allergies in a strategic way. The following chapters will provide food service establishments with helpful tips and processes to assist them in building the knowledge, skills, and abilities of food service employees to be able to communicate important information to their customers and provide them with a safe dining experience.

WHAT IS A FOOD ALLERGY
OR INTOLERANCE?

For years, scientists have argued about the true definition of allergies. Since this book covers more than just food allergies, following are related terms and their meanings.

- *Food allergy* refers to a particular type of response of the immune system in which the body produces what is called an allergic, or IgE, antibody to a food. (IgE, or immunoglobulin E, is a type of protein that works against a specific food.)[1]

- *Food intolerance* refers to an abnormal response to a food or additive, but it differs from an allergy in that it does not involve the immune system.[2]
- *Food sensitivity* is used as an umbrella term for food allergy, food intolerance, and other adverse reactions to food, unless they are psychological in origin.[3]
- *Food aversion* means "dislike and avoidance of a particular food for purely psychological reasons."[4]
- *Anaphylaxis* is a severe reaction to an allergen that can cause itching, fainting, and in some cases death.[5]
- *Celiac disease* is a chronic inflammatory disorder of the small intestine in genetically susceptible individuals. Ingesting certain proteins, commonly referred to as "gluten" that is naturally present in some cereal grains, triggers it.[6]

FACTS AND STATISTICS

The following facts and statistics will provide a better understanding of how serious food allergies are becoming. This information is from the 2008 Food Allergy Facts and Statistics prepared by the Food Allergy & Anaphylaxis Network:

- There are more than 12 million Americans who have a food allergy, which represents 1 in 25, or 4% of the population.
- Food allergy is believed to be the leading cause of anaphylaxis outside the hospital setting; causing an estimated 50,000 emergency room visits each year.
- Each year in the United States, it is estimated that approximately 150 to 200 people die due to a food allergy reaction. Death can be sudden, occurring within minutes. One of the reasons for this is that people did not know they were allergic to a specific food or did not have a written plan from their doctor for preventing and treating reactions.
- Strict avoidance of the food allergen, and early recognition and management of allergic reactions to food are important measures to prevent serious consequences.
- There is no cure for a food allergy.

DO FOOD ALLERGIES AFFECT
MORE CHILDREN THAN ADULTS?

There are reports that indicate that more children have a food allergy than adults. In October 2008, the U.S. Department of Health and Human Services published a report titled "Food Allergy Among U.S. Children: Trends in Prevalence and Hospitalization." The report states that 4 out of every 100 children have a food allergy and that food allergies affect some ethnic groups differently. Here are some of the key findings from the report:

- From 1997 to 2007, the prevalence of reported food allergy increased 18% among children under age 18.
- From 2004 to 2006, there were approximately 9,500 hospital discharges per year with diagnosis related to food allergy among children under age 18.
- In 2007, approximately 3 million children under the age of 18 years (3.9%) were reported to have a food or digestive allergy in the previous 12 months.
- Children with a food allergy are 2 to 4 times more likely to have other related conditions such as asthma and other allergies, compared with children without food allergies.
- The incidence of food allergy is highest in young children: 1 in 17 under the age of 3.

Based on another report written by Dr. Vaishali Mankad and A. Wesley Burks, food allergies affect up to 6% of young children and 3.5% of adults in the United States. Today, it is not uncommon to know a family member, neighbor, or friend affected by a food allergy.[7]

While presenting at the 2009 FAAN Teen Event in Arlington, Virginia, I had the opportunity to talk to teens about their allergies. Out of 110 teens, 75% had asthma and 50% of those kids had multiple allergies. From my kitchen experience, I have also noticed an increase in food allergy requests that are due to parents requesting meals for their children with food allergies and not themselves.

FOOD ALLERGY STATISTICS FROM OTHER COUNTRIES

Food allergies do not only affect the American population but also affect people around the world. People in other countries are not only allergic to the top eight food allergens but may be allergic to other foods such as beef, chicken, corn, fruits, rice, and sesame seeds, just to name a few. The top food allergens may be different for each country. This is based on the theory that the most common foods eaten by a culture leads to the development of allergies to these foods. It is estimated that 3% to 4% of the world's population are affected by food allergies.[8]

The United States is not the only country leading the charge on food allergy awareness, education, and research. Australia, Canada, Hong Kong, Japan, and United Kingdom have also been dealing with food allergies. The following statistics highlight the growing concern for continuing the efforts to learn more about food allergies and how we can help the families that cope with them.

AUSTRALIA

The following statistics are provided by Anaphylaxis Australia, Inc., a nonprofit Australian charity that provides support to health and teaching professionals, members of the food industry, and all who are touched by life-threatening allergies.

- Five percent of Australian children will develop a food allergy by school age.
- One percent of Australian adults currently have a food allergy.
- There is evidence that food allergy has increased in Australia and other countries in the last decade.
- Peanut allergy is estimated to affect 2% to 3% of children by school age.
- In 80 percent of children with peanut allergy, it remains a life-long problem.[9]

Australia also has startling figures about hospital visits.

- Hospital admissions for anaphylaxis have doubled over the 12-year period from 1995 to 2007.
- Of these admissions, rates for food-induced anaphylaxis in children 0 to 4 years have increased fivefold.
- The rates for children ages 5 to 14 years old have increased fourfold.[10]

CANADA

In a recent article titled "Canadian Data Are In" published in the spring 2010 issue of *Allergic Living*, Dr. Moshe Ben-Shoshan presented new data that showed an increase in "probable" peanut and tree nut allergies that were higher than the U.S. rate. The term "probable" is used to identify those people with a history of food allergy or have been diagnosed by a doctor.

- Children (probable allergy)
    - Peanut, 1.68%
    - Tree nuts, 1.59%
    - Fish, 0.18%
    - Shellfish, 0.5%
    - Sesame, 0.23%
- Adult (probable allergy)
    - Peanut, 0.71%
    - Tree nuts, 1%
    - Fish, 0.56%
    - Shellfish, 1.69%
    - Sesame, 0.05%
- Approximately 1.3 million Canadians live with foods allergies, representing 4% of the total population.

HONG KONG

These statistics are from a study of approximately 325,000 preschoolers 2 to 7 years of age.[11]

- Beef, 0.52%
- Cow's milk, 0.46%
- Crustacean, 1.28%

- Egg, 0.73%
- Fish, 0.32%
- Peanut, 0.65%
- Tree nuts, 0.41%

JAPAN

According to an article written June 21, 2009, and posted by the Japan Offspring Fund titled, "Better Food Allergy Labeling Needed," the numbers of children with food allergy problems are increasing in Japan. The lists of food allergens that must be listed on a food label are wheat, soba (buckwheat) egg, milk, and peanuts. There are 20 more common allergens that are recommended for food labeling and are usually placed below the ingredient statement. These include beef, chicken, pork, shellfish (abalone, shrimp, crab), fish (fish roe, fish eggs, salmon, mackerel), fruit (apple, banana, orange, kiwi fruit, peach), mushroom, soybeans, walnut, and yam.[12]

A study by the Ministry of Health, Labor and Welfare reported that

- Seven percent of the population (8.75 million) had some form of food allergy
- Among patients who visited hospitals with a food allergy
  - 80% were children
  - 9% were adults
- 11% of the patients had experienced a life-threatening anaphylaxis shock

UNITED KINGDOM

- Up to 2 people in every 100 in the United Kingdom have a diagnosed food allergy, and an additional 1 person in 100 has an intolerance to gluten. This is equal to a total of 1.5 million people.
- About 10 deaths a year due to food allergy are reported.
- Repeated reactions are seen in about 50% of those with a diagnosed food allergy, despite their efforts to avoid the foods to which they react.[13]

GLOBAL MARKET RESEARCH REPORT

A landmark global research sponsored and funded exclusively by AllergyFree Passport® and GlutenFree Passport® titled "Understanding Gluten and Allergen-Free Experiences of Guests & Hospitality Worldwide" was conducted in 2008. This detailed report shows the increase of food allergies worldwide and includes the perception of the food-allergic customer and the food service industry on their view of food allergy awareness.

Here are some of the key findings from this report:

- Peanut, tree nut, eggs, and milk are the most common foods that cause an allergy reaction (Figure 1.2).
- Of 350 respondents, 49% of children under the age of 5 have a food allergy (Figure 1.3).
- Families surveyed have been managing food allergies for as long as 5 years (refer to Figure 1.3).
- The biggest eating challenges include finding safe foods to eat, preparing meals, and ensuring balanced and nutritious diets.
- The daily stress of managing food allergies is due to:
  - Diligent reading of food labels
  - Concerns about cross-contamination
  - Feeling of being alone and lack of understanding
  - Fear of having a life-threatening reaction[14]
- There is a need for improvement associated with gluten and allergen-free living in the following areas (Figure 1.4):
  - Expanded training for food service providers
  - A wider selection of better tasting products
  - Gluten and allergen-free awareness initiatives
- Sixty-two percent of the hospitality and food service respondents consider gluten- and allergen-free guests as a new and profitable customer segment translating into potential increased revenue streams for food service providers.[15]
- There is a tremendous gap in the perspectives of understanding special diets between the guests and hospitality, consumers, and businesses.
- It indicates that consumers believe less than 10% of eating establishments have a very good or good understanding of gluten- and allergen-free diets (Figure 1.5).

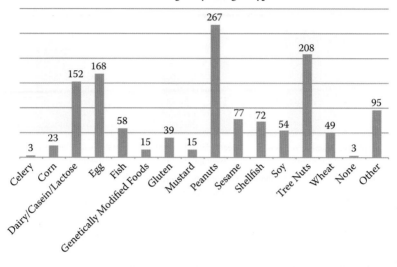

FIGURE 1.2

FOOD ALLERGIES BY ALLERGEN TYPE.

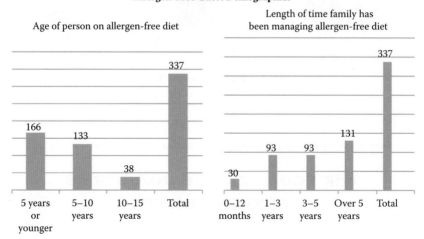

FIGURE 1.3

ALLERGEN-FREE GUEST DEMOGRAPHICS.

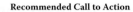

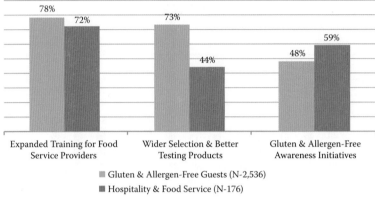

FIGURE 1.4

RECOMMENDED CALL TO ACTION.

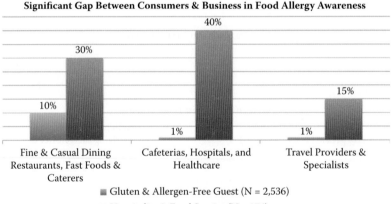

FIGURE 1.5

SIGNIFICANT GAP BETWEEN CONSUMERS AND BUSINESS IN FOOD ALLERGY AWARENESS.

THE FOOD SERVICE INDUSTRY'S RESPONSIBILITY

Is the food service industry doing enough? Based on AllergyFree Passport's report, there is still a long way to go considering what the customers had to say. My wife, Mary, and I have had the opportunity to travel extensively throughout the United States over the last 7 years and conducted our own study of the food service industry's knowledge, skills, and abilities on handling food-allergy requests. We visited the following cities and asked basic food allergy questions: Las Vegas and Reno, Nevada; Copper Mountain, Boulder, and Denver, Colorado; Chicago, Illinois; Providence, Rhode Island; Arlington, Virginia; Portland, Oregon; and Seattle, Washington. There was not one specific city that did better than the others, but we saw the biggest improvement in Las Vegas. We asked the following questions:

- Do you take care of guests with food allergies?
- Do you have a process for handling food-allergy requests?
- Do you have a special menu for people with special diets?
- I have a food allergy to milk. Can you safely make anything for me to eat?
- Can you make any substitutions on this menu for items containing milk?
- Do you have any desserts without milk as an ingredient?

I can tell you that in the beginning it was really bad. Many places, even the fine dining restaurants, did not even know what a food allergy was, let alone having a process in place. I remember visiting an upscale steakhouse in Las Vegas where we were told that they *would not* serve us and we would have to eat somewhere else.

When it came to special menus, there were none at all. At least now, some of the chain restaurants, including Bonefish Grill, Carrabba's Italian Grill, On The Border, Outback Steakhouse, P.F. Chang's, and Ruby Tuesday's, offer gluten-free menu options.

Avoiding milk and trying to get substitutions was another challenge. I rarely ever talked to a chef or manager about my dietary concerns and when I did, many of them did not know the ingredients in their own menu items or about cross-contact. Many of the servers did not even know that there was milk in half-and-half. Even today, I can hardly get a dessert that doesn't contain milk. I am lucky I do not eat dessert very often and do not have a severe food allergy.

I do have to say, food allergy awareness in restaurants has improved over the last seven years. On return trips to Las Vegas, restaurants have been willing to accommodate food allergy and special dietary requests. Many restaurants either had a process in place or had a statement on the menu to notify management if you had a food allergy or special diet. I noticed that chefs were more willing to make substitutions and the options were more creative and tasty.

This does not mean the food service industry is ready to handle all food allergy requests, but it does show that the industry is starting to take them more seriously. The next step is education. The industry needs to learn more about how food allergies work, the symptoms of a food allergy reaction, how they can be treated, and what steps need to be taken to provide safe menu options that are healthy, nutritious, and tasty.

HOW DO FOOD ALLERGIC
REACTIONS WORK?

When a food is digested for the first time, it causes the body to produce the food-specific IgE antibody that then attaches to the *mast cells* and *basophiles*, which are found in all body tissue. Mast cells are large granule-containing cells found in areas of the body that are typical sites for allergic reactions, such as the nose, throat, lungs, skin, and gastrointestinal (GI) tract. Basophiles are white blood cells that contribute to inflammatory reactions. Once the food is digested again, it interacts with food-specific IgE on the surface of the mast cells and causes the cells to release chemicals such as histamine. The histamines inside the resting mast cells look like small granules under the microscope, so the process of releasing the chemicals is called degranulation (see Figure 1.6).[16]

Histamine and the other chemicals released by mast cells are called mediators because they bring about or mediate changes in the body. These mediators contain 10 or more different substances, and each one has its own effect on the body. Some make the blood vessels open out, others make them more leaky so that blood escapes through the vessel walls. This leakage can cause inflammation and swelling of the tissues.[17]

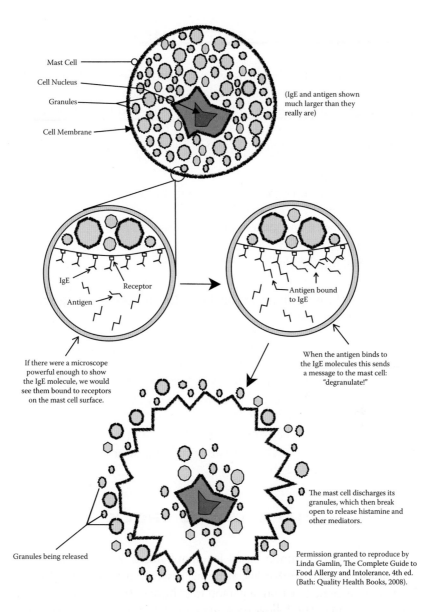

Mast Cell

Cell Nucleus

Granules

Cell Membrane

(IgE and antigen shown much larger than they really are)

IgE

Receptor

Antigen

Antigen bound to IgE

If there were a microscope powerful enough to show the IgE molecule, we would see them bound to receptors on the mast cell surface.

When the antigen binds to the IgE molecules this sends a message to the mast cell: "degranulate!"

The mast cell discharges its granules, which then break open to release histamine and other mediators.

Granules being released

Permission granted to reproduce by Linda Gamlin, The Complete Guide to Food Allergy and Intolerance, 4th ed. (Bath: Quality Health Books, 2008).

FIGURE 1.6
FOOD ALLERGY REACTION IN THE MAST CELL.

FOOD ALLERGY SYMPTOMS

A food allergic reaction happens when the body does not recognize the protein as safe or can no longer tolerate the allergen. Some reactions to food allergens can be severe to life threatening, and take place within a few minutes or it could take as long as 2 hours to happen. The most common signs and symptoms of a food allergy include:

- Hives, itching, or skin rash
- Swelling of the lips, face, tongue, and throat, or other parts of the body
- Wheezing, nasal congestion, or trouble breathing
- Abdominal pain, diarrhea, nausea, or vomiting
- Dizziness, lightheadedness, or fainting

The process of eating and digesting food also affects the timing and the location of a reaction.

- If a person is allergic to a particular food, he or she may first feel itching in the mouth as the food is first eaten.
- After the food is digested in the stomach, it may cause GI symptoms.
- When the food allergen enters and travels through the bloodstream, it may cause blood pressure to drop.
- As the allergen reaches the skin, it may cause hives or eczema.
- When the allergen reaches the throat or lungs, it may cause throat tightness and trouble breathing.[18]

ANAPHYLACTIC SHOCK

Today, the most common cases for anaphylactic reations are foods, aspirin-like drugs, antibiotics, stinging insects, and latex products.[19] In an anaphylactic reaction, a person may have extreme versions of the same symptoms. The following signs and symptoms characterize this type of reaction:

- Swelling of the tongue and throat to where it is impossible to breath
- Shock, with a severe drop in blood pressure
- Rapid, irregular pulse

- Loss of consciousness
- Death

When these events occur, the person having the reaction will need medical assistance quickly. They need to receive a shot of adrenaline from an epinephrine pen, also called an epipen. This will quickly reduce the amount of histamines in the body, long enough to allow the person to get life-saving medical assistance. Studies have shown that early administration of epinephrine is key to successfully treating anaphylactic reactions.[20]

HOW ALLERGENS ARE INTRODUCED TO THE BODY

Food allergens are introduced to the body in three ways: ingestion, contact, or inhalation.

- *Ingestion* is the most common way for a person with food allergies to come in contact with an offending food. This usually happens when the person eats a food that has a hidden food allergen in the ingredients.
- *Contact* happens when a person with a food allergy is touched by someone that has come in contact with an offending food or the person touches something (i.e., table, chair, utensil, plate, etc.) that has an offending protein residue leftover from improper cleaning and sanitizing procedures.
- *Inhalation* happens when a person with a food allergy inhales an airborne allergen from peanuts or nuts being roasted in an open vending area or from vapors from steaming fish or shrimp in a restaurant.

METHODS OF ALLERGEN INTRODUCTION INTO FOOD

Since many food allergic consumers do not make all of their food from scratch, there are many ways that a food allergen can be present in foods they purchase at the grocery store or in restaurants.

- *Cross-contact* happens when an item comes in contact with a potential allergen in food preparation at home or in a restaurant. This can happen when utensils, pots, pans, or hands are not properly washed and sanitized between food preparations.
- *Residues* are food particles left over from manufacturing processes and are not listed on the ingredient label. An example is not properly cleaning production lines between the preparations of food containing certain allergens and ones that do not contain these allergens.
- *By-products* are food items produced from another food's manufacturing process and are not properly listed on the ingredient label. An example is casein or whey from milk that are added to a product and mistakenly not listed on the label.
- *Subingredients* are ingredients that are present in prepackaged foods that are added to another food and not listed on the label. This may happen when a food service location prepares its own products that are packaged for sale and but do not list all of the individual ingredients on the label.

Since accurate ingredient labeling is such a critical requirement to keep the food allergic customer safe, the Food and Drug Administration (FDA) established regulations to ensure that the food service industry had the proper guidelines to follow to ensure this took place. This will be discussed in more detail in Chapter 2.

TREATMENT FOR FOOD ALLERGY

Unfortunately, there is no cure for a food allergy. There is only strict avoidance of the offending food for life. To do this, the food-allergic person must read food labels and ingredient statements thoroughly to help identify potential allergens and their subingredients.

Many allergy-producing foods, such as milk, eggs, and peanuts, appear in many processed foods and restaurant menu items. Since the enactment of the Food Allergen Labeling and Consumer Protection Act of 2004 (FALCPA), it is easier for consumers to identify the top eight food allergens on food labels.

Minor food allergy reactions can be treated with an antihistamine, such as Benadryl®, but if someone in your establishment has a severe food allergy reaction, do not deny it, argue with the guest, or defend the restaurant—*you must notify management immediately and call 911.* This is the only way to make sure the customer gets the needed life-saving medical treatment. There have been reports of people having a second food allergy reaction, sometimes more severe, 24 to 48 hours after having the first reaction.

FOOD ALLERGIES TODAY

It is important to understand that in the early 1900s our world looked a lot different than it does now. There were more people living on farms and eating natural foods. There were few preservatives and no mass-produced foods. Chemicals and pesticides were not widely used and there was less pollution and environmental contaminates in the air. Could the increase in the use of preservatives, chemicals, and these other environmental changes have an affect on the increase of food allergies in the American population? This is still unknown, but there are many theories that try to answer this question.

FOOD ALLERGY THEORIES

Several theories have been put forth to attempt to explain the rise in food allergies. In an article published in the October–November 2006 issue of *Food Allergy News* titled "Are Food Allergies on the Rise?" two doctors wrote about the most recent theories.

The "hygiene hypothesis," first proposed by British researcher Dr. David Stachan in 1989, suggests that exposure to certain germs and infections early in life are important in training the immune system to do what it is intended to do: recognize foreign threats to the body. The American way of life, cleanliness and obsession, with hygiene has skewed the immune system toward the development of allergic diseases.[21] Evidence supporting this theory is that allergies are more common in developed countries and less common in children that grow up on farms, attend daycare in early life, and who have multiple older siblings. Evidence refuting this theory is that some of the highest rates of asthma and allergies are in the inner city where hygiene is often no better than in undeveloped countries.

Another theory is the introduction of foods too early in a baby's diet, before the immune system is mature enough to handle them. This could occur through breastfeeding or exposure to processed foods that have hidden allergens.[22] This would support the research that states over the last three decades the number of people with allergies has increased in developed and developing countries, but not in under-developed countries.

The "detection bias" theory suggests that doctors are more aware of food allergies and are better able to diagnose it. Some suggest that food allergies were just as common in the past as they are now, but most experts do not share this view and believe that there is a true increase in food allergies.

Dr. Thomas Platt-Mills has proposed another theory called the "Couch Potato Theory." He thinks that the sedentary afterschool lifestyles of modern children (no outdoor play, lying on carpets or rugs, and watch-ing television or computer screens) allows children to spend more time indoors in poorly ventilated homes and apartments. Inner-city children often stay indoors after school due to violent neighborhoods. These homes may be loaded with indoor allergens, such as dust mites, molds, pets, and cockroaches, which in turn lead to increased allergy sensitization and asthma. This lifestyle also can lead to obesity in chil-dren where recent studies have shown a relationship between asthma and obese children.[23] In another study, Dr. Carlos Camargo studied 16,862 children ages nine to fourteen years of age and found that asthma was more prevalent in overweight children.[24]

A more recent theory is the "microflora hypothesis." This was spawned because some researchers believe that the hygiene hypothesis did not explain why inner-city children living in poor hygienic conditions have the highest rates of asthma in the world or why residents of clean moun-tain air have experienced the asthma and allergy epidemic as well. The microflora hypothesis proposes that the increase in allergies are due to a combination of overuse of antibiotics in infancy and early childhood, distruction of friendly bacteria in the intestinal tract, and a dramatic change in maternal and infant diet in the Westernized societies.[25]

What I find interesting about the antibiotic theory is that everytime I went to the doctor while I was growing up, it seemed like they would prescribe antibiotics. I would get sick more often back then. Since I have been married to my lovely and very healthy wife, Mary, I am much healthier. Now, when I get sick, which is not often, I do not take antibiotics unless I have to. This is because Mary always tells me to "stick it out" when I get sick and let the body do its job naturally. Mary rarely gets sick and when she does, she will not take antibiotics unless it is life or death. I have met parents that also believe that the increase of antibiotic use has led to their children getting allergies or autism. Unfortuately, this is only a theory and there is need for more study by the medical field.

CHAPTER IN REVIEW

There is no doubt that food allergies are on the rise in America and around the world and there is a need for further research. What we do know is that a food allergy is an autoimmune system response to a specific food and a reaction can be severe to life threatening. There is currently no cure for a food allergy, only complete avoidance of the food for life. Antihistamines and epinephrine are two types of medication that can help slow down a reaction. If someone has a severe food allergic reaction, he or she should take an ejection of epinephrine and seek medical help immediately because a second reaction could occur within 24 to 48 hours of the first reaction. Finally, there are plenty of theories that try to explain the increase in food allergies over the years, but the bottom line is that food allergies are not going away and the food service industry should take them seriously because they are real.

ENDNOTES

1. U.S. Department of Health and Human Services, "Food Allergy. An Overview" (Washington, D.C.: GPO, 2004), 2.
2. Jonathan Brostoff and Linda Gamlin, *The Complete Guide to Food Allergy and Intolerance*, 4th ed. (Bath: Quality Health Books, 2008), 12.
3. Ibid., 13.

4. Ibid., 12.
5. U.S. Department of Health and Human Services, 31.
6. U.S. Food and Drug Administration, "Questions and Answers on the Gluten-Free Labeling Proposed Rule" (Washington, D.C.: GPO, 2007).
7. Vaishali S. Mankad, MD and A. Wesley Burks, MD, "Are Food Allergies on the Rise?" *Food Allergy News* 16, no. 1 (2006): 1.
8. Kim Koeller, *Understanding Gluten and Allergen-Free Experiences of Guests & Hospitality Worldwide* (Chicago: AllergyFree Passport, 2008), 59.
9. Anaphylaxis Australia, "Food Allergy Fast Facts," http://www.allergyfacts.org.au/
10. Australasian Society of Clinical Immunology & Allergy, "The Economic Impact of Allergic Disease in Australia: Not to Be Sneezed At," November 13, 2007, 32.
11. T. F. Leung et al., "Parent reported adverse food reactions in Hong Kong Chinese preschoolers: epidemiology, clinical spectrum and risk factors," *Pediatric Allergy Immunology* 20, no. 4 (2009): 339–346.
12. Japan Offspring Fund, "Better Food Allergy Labeling Needed," June 21, 2009, http://japanoffspringfund.wordpress.com/2009/06/21/food-allergy-labelling/
13. Food Standards Agency Strategic Plan 2005–2010: "Putting Consumers First," p. 16, http://www.food.gov.uk/multimedia/pdfs/stratplan0510.pdf
14. AllergyFree Passport® May 2007: Kids with Food Allergies, "Challenges Among Food Allergic Children," 1.
15. Koeller, 11.
16. Brostoff and Gamlin, 72.
17. Ibid.
18. U.S. Department of Health and Human Services, 4.
19. Paul J. Hannaway, MD, *On the Nature of Food Allergy* (Marblehead, MA: Lighthouse Press, 2007), 45.
20. The Food Allergy & Anaphylaxis Network, "Food Allergy Facts and Statistics," 2008, http://www.foodallergy.org
21. Mankad and Burks, 9.
22. Ibid.
23. Hannaway, 22.
24. Ibid.
25. Ibid., 24.

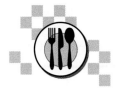

CHAPTER 2

Major Food Allergens Revealed

In the past it was very difficult for consumers to know if there were hidden food allergens in manufactured foods. To help consumers, the U.S. Food and Drug Administration (FDA) spent years working with food manufacturers, food allergy associations, and advocates to develop a law that would help identify the major food allergens in processed foods. This work created the Food Allergen Labeling and Consumer Protection Act. In this chapter we will review the provisions of the act, consumer advisory statements that have caused significant confusion and concern for the food allergic consumer and chefs alike, how manufacturing practices have changed leading up to the act, and how the act has affected changes to the Food Code and state regulations.

FOOD ALLERGEN LABELING AND CONSUMER PROTECTION ACT

In August 2004, the Food Allergen Labeling and Consumer Protection Act (FALCPA) was passed. By proper food labeling of allergens, this comprehensive food labeling law was designed to ensure those individuals with food allergies and other food-related concerns could easily and accurately identify food ingredients that may cause a reaction.

Even though the act was passed in 2004, it was not until January 1, 2006, that manufacturers had to have their labels compliant with the act's guidelines.

The FALCPA requirements:

- Ingredient labels are required to list the eight major food allergens in plain English. The eight allergens are milk, eggs, fish, shellfish, tree nuts, peanuts, soy, and wheat.
- Companies indicate the food allergens on their labels in two ways:
  - By placing the word "Contains" followed by the name of the food source from which the major food allergen is derived (e.g., "Contains egg and milk").
  - By placing the common or usual name of the allergen in the list of ingredients followed in parentheses by the name of the food source from which the allergen is derived (e.g., "natural flavoring [eggs, milk, soy]").
- The name of the allergen needs to appear only once in the ingredient statement. For example, a product that contains both milk and milk-derived ingredients, such as whey, would be labeled as follows: "milk, sodium caseinate, whey" or "natural flavor (milk), sodium caseinate, whey."
- In the case of nuts and seafood, the specific type of nut (e.g., walnut, almond, cashew) or species of fish (e.g., tuna, salmon) or shellfish (shrimp, crab, lobster) should be specified.
- It applies to all packaged foods (except meat, poultry, and certain egg products) sold in the United States.[1]

USDA FOOD ALLERGEN LABELING STATEMENT

FALCPA applies to packaged foods subject to FDA regulation, including foods both domestically manufactured and imported. That includes all foods, except meat, poultry, and egg products regulated by the U.S. Department of Agriculture's (USDA) Food Safety and Inspection Service (FSIS). To be consistent with FALCPA, FSIS is undertaking rulemaking to adopt the FALCPA requirements for the products it regulates. Meanwhile, meat, poultry, and egg products manufacturers may voluntarily add food allergen statements to their labels.[2]

CONSUMER ADVISORY STATEMENTS

With the FALCPA, there was now a law to help consumers with food allergies identify the foods that could make them sick. The food allergy community was very happy with the FALCPA, but there was now a new problem. Food manufacturers started to use "Consumer Advisory Statements" on many of their prepackaged foods with the following statements: "may contain," "processed in a plant," or "manufactured on shared lines." Foods that were once considered safe now contained one of these new statements. Why did the manufacturing companies start this labeling practice?

Most of the companies did this to advise the consumer of the possibility of potential allergens that may be present in their foods. Since manufacturers do not test every product for food allergens and cleaning processes are not a 100% guarantee that food allergens were removed from equipment, companies wanted to protect themselves from any lawsuits for mislabeling their products. This may have provided them with a sense of security but it just caused additional hardship on their consumers.

In 2006, the Food Allergy & Anaphylaxis Network (FAAN) published an article titled "Consumers Perspective: New Labeling Issues" describing consumers' issues with the use of advisory statements. FAAN says, "We have received an unprecedented number of calls and e-mails from members who are concerned about the proliferation of warning statements on products they have previously been using." The article goes on to provide comments from its members:

- "I have a child with multiple, severe allergies to foods including soy, nuts, and peanuts. Approximately 25% of the foods that I used to buy now have vague, unhelpful statements such as 'processed in a plant with soy, fish, peanuts,' etc. These labels now appear on everything from catsup, cream cheese, and jelly to vitamins. Either they are over-labeling, or don't use good food manufacturing practices."
- "I just bought a snack food for my 12-year-old with peanut and tree nut allergies. The package has this disclaimer—ALLERGEN INFORMATION: Good manufacturing practices (GMP) used to

segregate ingredients in a facility that also processes peanuts, tree nut, milk, soy, shellfish, and wheat ingredients.' How does one interpret this kind of information?"[3]

Even though these new statements have been difficult on the consumer, they are still visible on today's labels.

During this period, I remember receiving calls from concerned parents about these new statements. They were wondering if the foods that they had previously eaten at our restaurants were still safe. To assist our guests with this information we started reviewing our food labels to see which ones changed. In reviewing the food labels, we found many of the labels had these new advisory statements. We contacted our vendors to discuss the changes and to have them provide us with any updated food allergen statements. We were informed that this was their new policy but it did not change their current good manufacturing practices. This was very time consuming but necessary to provide our guests with the most up-to-date information. When a guest asked about ingredient statements, we would read the information off the label or refer them to the manufacturing company.

In January 2009, the FDA published an article titled, "Food Allergies: Reducing the Risk" where the report discussed current food labeling issues. It states that on September 16, 2008, the FDA held a public hearing to determine how manufacturers use advisory labeling for food allergens and to evaluate how consumers interpret different advisory labeling statements. The article states that consumer advisory statements have limited the variety of packaged foods that the food allergic consumer could purchase. The purpose of the statements was to inform the consumer of the possibility that a manufactured food could contain or have been contaminated by an allergen during production. Manufactured foods may be contaminated or come in contact (cross-contact) with an allergen during:

- Harvesting
- Transportation
- Manufacturing
- Processing
- Storage[4]

Many food manufacturers follow good manufacturing practices and try to prevent cross-contact through the use of segregating allergenic products, dedicated facilities, and dedicated production lines.

Before Hazard Analysis Critical Control Points (HACCP), the food service industry relied on the general sanitation requirements established by the FDA called the Good Manufacturing Practice Regulations and testing of finished products to remain in compliance with FDA requirements.

A BRIEF HISTORY OF GOOD MANUFACTURING PRACTICE (GMP) REGULATIONS

Since the enactment of the Food, Drug, and Cosmetic Act in 1938, the guidelines for manufacturing processes were very vague and not easily enforced by the U.S. Department of Agriculture. There were two particular sections of the Food, Drug, and Cosmetic Act that were extremely vague. There were specific provisions of the law that directly related to conditions in a facility where food was being manufactured. These provisions were unlike other parts that related to the conditions of a facility where food is produced or stored. Thus, instead of having to prove that the food was adulterated, unsanitary conditions were considered sufficient to show that the food might have been adulterated.[5]

In the mid-1960s the FDA began drafting new GMP regulations. The objective of the GMP regulations was to describe general rules for maintaining sanitary conditions that must be followed by all food-processing facilities to ensure that statutory requirements were met.[6]

When the final GMP regulations were completed they were still very broad. They did not specify what exactly a facility must do to comply. This made it difficult for the FDA to enforce. To address this issue, the FDA tried to develop industry-specific GMPs but these revisions were unrealistic. Instead, the FDA decided to improve the general GMPs. The additional revision was finalized in 1986 (see Figure 2.1).

FIGURE 2.1

HISTORICAL TIMELINE FOR GOOD MANUFACTURING PRACTICES.

Date	Event
1906	The Bureau of Chemistry passes the 1906 Pure Food and Drugs Act, prohibiting interstate commerce in misbranded and adulterated foods, drinks, and drugs.
1933	The Food and Drug Administration (FDA) recommends revising the 1906 Pure Food and Drugs Act.
1938	FDA passes the 1938 Federal Food, Drug, and Cosmetics (FD&C) Act, which provides identity and quality standards for food.
Mid-1960s	FDA decides to clarify the FD&C Act through Good Manufacturing Practice (GMP) regulations.
1968	FDA proposes food GMP regulations.
1969	FDA finalizes food GMP regulations.
Early 1970s	FDA considers implementing industry-specific regulations.
Late 1970s	FDA decides to revise the general GMPs rather than adopting industry-specific GMPs.
1986	FDA publishes revised food GMPs.
2002	FDA forms Food GMP Modernization Working Group.
2004	FDA announces efforts to modernize food GMPs.

Source: Dunkelberger, 1995; FDA, 1981b.

The current GMPs consist of seven subparts, two of which were omitted from the report. Here is a brief description of the provisions:

- 1.2.1 General Provisions included term definitions, employee personal hygiene, food safety education and training, and criteria for determining adulteration of foods.
- 1.2.2 Buildings and Facilities included requirements for adequate maintenance, layout, and operations of food-processing plants, sanitary operations of physical facilities, equipment, and utensils to protect against food contamination. The section also briefly addressed pest control and cleaning of various food contact surfaces and cleaning frequency.
- 1.2.3 Equipment described the requirements and expectations for the design, construction, and maintenance of equipment and utensils so as to ensure sanitary conditions.
- 1.2.4 Production and Process Controls listed general sanitation processes and controls necessary to ensure that food was suitable for human consumption. It addressed the monitoring of physical factors (critical control points), such as time, temperature, humidity, pH, flow rate, and acidification.
- 1.2.5 Defect Action Levels (DALs), the last subpart, defined the maximum defect action levels for a defect that is natural or unavoidable even when foods are produced under current GMPs as set out in the other sections of the regulations.[7]

The requirements provided clear guidelines of what a facility must do to comply but were made general enough to allow many manufacturers the flexibility to implement the requirements that would best meet their needs.

NOTICE TO MANUFACTURERS

Even with these guidelines, the FDA received reports every year of consumers who had experienced illness or adverse reactions to foods that contained allergenic substances. These exposures occurred because the allergen in the food was not declared on the package label. So on June 10, 1996, the FDA sent an "allergy warning letter" to all manufacturers. In this letter, it highlighted the 1938 Food, Drug, and Cosmetic Act requirements concerning proper food labeling. A number of the incidents related to two of the sections that many manufacturers were misinterpreting.

- Section 403(i) of the act provides that spices, flavorings, and colorings may be declared collectively without naming each one.
- Regulation (21 CFR 101.100(a)(3)) exempts ingredient declaration for incidental additives, such as processing aids, that are present in a food at insignificant levels and that do not have a technical or functional effect in the finished food.

The other misinterpretation of the act was the insignificant amount of an allergenic ingredient. Since it was not a main ingredient in the food and was used as a processing agent, flavoring, or spice, many manufacturers were not indicating this on their labels. Some manufacturers maintained that some allergens that were used as processing aids qualified for this exemption, but the FDA never considered food allergens eligible for this exemption. There was sufficient evidence suggesting that some allergens could cause serious allergic reactions in some individuals upon eating a very small amount of the allergen.

At that time, the FDA had not formally defined "allergens," but it provided examples of foods that were among the most commonly known to cause an allergic reaction. These, of course were the top eight foods. This policy statement dealing with foods derived from new plant varieties was published in the *Federal Register* of May 29, 1992.[8]

The FDA did ask the manufacturers to take three additional steps:

- First, examine their product formulations for ingredients and processing aids that contain known allergens that they may have considered to be exempt and to declare the presence of these ingredients by name and place them on the ingredient statement.
- Second, voluntarily declare allergenic ingredients of a color, flavor, or spice by simply naming it on the ingredient label.
- Third, the FDA was aware of certain manufacturers voluntarily labeling their products with the statement "may contain i.e., egg, milk, etc." The FDA advised that such precautionary labeling should not be used

instead of adhering to the current GMPs. The manufacturers should take all the steps necessary to eliminate cross-contamination and to ensure the absence of the allergenic food.[9]

STATEMENT OF POLICY FOR LABELING AND PREVENTING CROSS-CONTACT

In April 2001, the Food and Drug Administration came out with Sec. 555.250 "Statement of Policy for Labeling and Preventing Cross-Contact of Common Food Allergens." This policy had one very substantial requirement called "Practices Used to Prevent Potential Allergen Cross-Contact." This policy states:

> Allergens may be unintentionally added to food as a result of practices such as improper rework addition, product carry-over due to the use of common equipment and production sequencing, or the presence of an allergenic product above exposed product lines. Such practices with respect to allergenic substances may be unsanitary conditions that may render food injurious to health and adulterate the product under section 402(a)(4) of the Act [21 U.S.C. 342(a)(4)].[10]

FOOD GOOD MANUFACTURING PRACTICES MODERNIZATION WORKING GROUP

In July 2002, the FDA formed a Food Good Manufacturing Practices Modernization Working Group to examine the effectiveness of current food GMPs given the many changes that have occurred in the food industry since 1986. The Working Group researched the impact of food GMPs on food safety and the impact of revised regulations. Part of the group's effort was to find out which elements of the food GMPs are critical to retain and which should be improved.

From the group's recommendations, the FDA established that food manufacturers who handle any of the eight major food allergens should be required to develop, adopt, and update as necessary, an allergen control plan. The requirements of the plan included six key areas of control:

- Training of processing and supervisory personnel
- Segregation of food allergens during storage and handling
- Validated cleaning procedures for food contact equipment
- Prevention of cross-contact by food allergens during food processing (e.g., by scheduling production runs, control or rework, or using dedicated production lines)
- Product labeling review, use, and control
- Supplier controls for ingredients and labels

In addition, food-manufacturing establishments should be required to maintain a copy of the allergen control plan at the processing facilities. The plan should be updated when changes to ingredients, products, processing, or labeling occur.[11] Figure 2.2 shows examples of points in the manufacturing process where cross-contact can occur and of the control practices used by manufacturers. These recommendations were extremely important and set the framework for the Food Allergen Labeling and Consumer Protection Act.

TESTING FOR FOOD ALLERGENS

Manufacturing companies can test their products for specific food allergens by using specially designed test kits or sending samples of their products to reputable companies such as Silliker® Food Safety and Quality Solutions, which provide testing for many common food allergens. The ELISA (enzyme-linked immunosorbent assay) is commonly used to test for gluten.

THE FOOD AND DRUG
ADMINISTRATION'S 2005 FOOD CODE

The FDA's Food Code is what the food service industry lives by, so it is important to understand how it applies to food allergy management. The Food Code applies to all establishments at the retail level that provide food directly to the public, including restaurants, grocery

FIGURE 2.2

MANUFACTURING PROCESSES WHERE CROSS-CONTACT CAN OCCUR.

Food Product Category	Specific Points Where Cross-Contact Can Occur	Examples of Control Practices Used
Bakery products	Mixers, shared equipment, packaging equipment, dividers, conveyors, ingredient scales, proofer, cooler, slicer, racks, piping, dough troughs, pans, belts, ovens, enrobing, freezer, changeovers, rounder, extruder, sheeter, baking room, crossed lines, shared storage containers, dough pump, dead spots, scoops, sifters, depositer, and sieves	Scheduling, sanitation, training, storage segregation, visual inspection, allergen testing, color-coding allergen products, push-through, equipment design, tarps under conveyors, labeling, vacuum, line separation, shields, distance, production layout, eliminate crossed lines, allergen profiling, scraping, segregated steam room for cleaning, color-code rework, dedicated areas, dedicated maintenance tools, and harmonization
Beverages	Filler, shared equipment, storage tanks, blending, pumps, lines, pasteurization, homogenization, liquefiers, and batch tanks	Sanitation, scheduling, allergen testing, visual inspection, and flushing

continued

FIGURE 2.2 (CONTINUED)
MANUFACTURING PROCESSES WHERE CROSS-CONTACT CAN OCCUR.

Food Product Category	Specific Points Where Cross-Contact Can Occur	Examples of Control Practices Used
Candy and confections	Enrober, packaging, panning, shared lines, coating, molding, belts, ovens, temper units, piping, refining, spraying systems, conveyors, and changeovers	Scheduling, sanitation, dedicated lines, flushing, wet cleaning where possible, segregation, dry cleaning, disassembly of equipment to clean, product formulation, labeling, dedicated equipment, wrap products prior to packaging, dedicated employees, inspection, allergen testing, and single-use storage bags
Cereals and pasta	Belts, mixers, particulates, packaging, shared lines, conveyors, scales, residue, piping, ovens, handling, rework, baking room, egg feeder, shared equipment, driers, shakers, sifters, crossed lines, reuse of storage containers, changeover, and reuse of frying oil	Sanitation, scheduling, separation, visual inspection, shielding, vacuum, dedication, eliminate cross-overs, pressure washing, disassembly of equipment for cleaning, flush with cornstarch, equipment design, and allergen testing

Food	Sources of cross-contact	Controls
Dairy products and substitutes	Shared equipment, fillers, blending, pasteurization, homogenization, storage tanks, shared lines, liquefiers, batch tanks, packaging equipment, and ingredient receiving.	Scheduling, sanitation, allergen testing, inspection, flushing, dedication, shields, separation, and supplier contact
Desserts	Shared equipment, fillers, pumps, storage tanks, lines, duct work, cooling systems, changeovers, fruit feeders, and varigators	Sanitation, scheduling, allergen testing, inspection, and production layout
Fish and fish products	Batter and breader equipment, freezer, fryer, packaging and conveyor belts	Scheduling, sanitation, prerequisites, filter oil, validation test, receipt of original containers at specific line assignments, equipment design, equipment flexibility, and inspection
Mixed dishes	Shared equipment, filler, mixer, conveyors, dead spots, and spice rooms	Sanitation, scheduling, equipment design, allergen testing, visual inspection, dedicated lines, and segregated storage

continued

FIGURE 2.2 (CONTINUED)

MANUFACTURING PROCESSES WHERE CROSS-CONTACT CAN OCCUR.

Food Product Category	Specific Points Where Cross-Contact Can Occur	Examples of Control Practices Used
Sauces, dips, gravies, and condiments	Piping, filler, mixer, scales, utensils, common tasks, spice room, shared lines, reused fryer oil, and conveyors	Sanitation, scheduling, allergen profiling, color-coding, elimination of dead spots, segregated storage, shielding, visual inspection, and labeling
Snack foods	Packaging, conveyors, belts, ovens, dryers, enrobers, mixers, shared equipment, crossed lines, reuse of storage containers, changeovers, dead spots, and reuse of fryer oil	Sanitation, visual inspection, equipment design, walls, scheduling, allergen testing, dedication, training, color-coding, segregated storage, eliminate cross-overs, and labeling
Soups	Spice rooms, dead spots, and shared lines	Scheduling, sanitation, separation, equipment design, and segregated storage

stores, supermarkets, hospitals, nursing homes, child care centers, and temporary food establishments. What is not commonly known is that the Food Code is a model code available for adoption by local, state, and other jurisdictions. Certain aspects of the law are open for interpretation by each state and can be used as a guideline when creating local laws.

You may have seen food allergy statements in a grocery store deli or on restaurant menus pop up over the last few years. This is because in 2005, after the FALCPA was established, the FDA updated the Food Code with new food allergen information including:

- A definition of "major food allergen" that is consistent with the definition in the FALCPA [Paragraph 1-201.10(B)].
- A new provision under Demonstration of Knowledge [Subparagraph 2-102.11)C)(9)] specifying that the person in charge of a food establishment shall have an understanding of the foods identified as major food allergens and the symptoms that a major food allergen could cause in a sensitive individual. This additional element is significant because nationally recognized certifiers of food managers who provide training and testing of such managers consult these elements when the certifiers routinely upgrade their training and testing programs.
- Integration of FALCPA's labeling provisions to reflect the additional requirements that apply to food that is packaged at the retail level [Subparagraph 3-602.11(B)(5)].[12]

In 2009, the Food Code was revised to expand the recommendations to all restaurant and food service employees. It is hoped that individual states will adopt the 2009 Food Code to help expand food allergy awareness to as many restaurants as possible.

STATE INITIATIVES

The Food and Drug Administration is not the only legislative body that has enacted food allergy laws. Over the past several years there have been numerous states that have enacted laws to protect children and teens in schools and the food allergic consumer in restaurants. The new

Advocacy section of FAAN's Web site includes current national and state issues and laws that have passed in recent years.

One of the most significant state laws passed was in Massachusetts. One of the articles states,

> On January 15, 2009, Governor Patrick of Massachusetts signed Senate Bill 2701 into law. This landmark legislation, the first of its kind in the U.S., calls on restaurants in Massachusetts to:
>
> - Display a food allergy poster in the restaurant staff area
> - Place a notice on menus of the customer's obligation to inform the server about any food allergies
> - Train food protection managers and persons in charge of restaurants on food allergy issues
>
> The Massachusetts legislation also allows restaurants to earn a "Food Allergy Friendly" designation from the Department of Public Health.[13]

Along with other proposed bills in New York, Connecticut, and Pennsylvania you should expect to see more states follow suit and adopt similar laws. This should only encourage you to learn more about food allergy safety, since your state may be drafting its own laws that will affect your establishment.

CHAPTER REVIEW

Since the early 20th century, the U.S. government has enacted laws to protect Americans from misleading information concerning food, drugs, and cosmetics that could do us harm. As our society moved further away from single-farmed foods to mass-produced, enhanced, manufactured foods, the Food and Drug Administration's Food Code had to change to adapt to the changing industry. By implementing Good Manufacturing Practices, Hazard Analysis Critical Control Point guidelines, and labeling standards the public has received safer foods to consume. With the rise of food allergy incidents in the last two decades, the FDA had to address this issue with the enactment of Food Allergen Labeling and Consumer Protection Act. FALCPA brought about safer GMPs and easier to read labels but not without cost to the food allergic consumer. New advisory statements reduced the quantity of foods they can eat and added a level of anxiety to their shopping experiences. Even though this is a good start to protect the food allergic consumer from potential life-threatening allergens, the law has a long way to go.

ENDNOTES

1. U.S. Food and Drug Administration, "Food Allergen Labeling and Consumer Protection Act of 2004 (Public Law 108-282, Title II)," http://www.fda.gov/Food/LabelingNutrition/FoodAllergensLabeling/ GuidanceComplianceRegulatoryInformation/ucm106187.htm
2. U.S. Department of Agriculture, "Get the Facts: New Food Allergen Labeling Law," http://www.fns.usda.gov/fdd/facts/nutrition/foodallergenfactsheet.pdf
3. The Food Allergy & Anaphylaxis Network, "Consumers Perspective: New Labeling Issues" Food Allergy Corporate Bulletin.
4. U.S. Food and Drug Administration, "Food Allergies: Reducing the Risks," http//www.fda.gov/consumer
5. U.S. Food and Drug Administration, "GMPs—Section One: Current Food Good Manufacturing Practices," http://www.fda.gov/Food/Guidance-ComplianceRegulatoryInformation/CurrentGoodManufacturingPractices-CGMPs/ucm110907.htm
6. GMPs—Section One: Current Food Good Manufacturing Practices.
7. Ibid.
8. U.S. Food and Drug Administration, "FDA Allergy Warning Letter," http://www.fda.gov/Food/LabelingNutrition/FoodAllergensLabeling/ GuidanceComplianceRegulatoryInformation/ucm106546.htm
9. Ibid.
10. U.S. Food and Drug Administration, "CPG Sec. 555.250 Statement of Policy for Labeling and Preventing Cross-contact of Common Food Allergens (New 4/2001)," http://www.fda.gov/ICECI/ComplianceManuals/ CompliancePolicyGuidanceManual/ucm074552.htm
11. Food CGMP Modernization Working Group, "Food CGMP Modernization—A Focus on Food Safety." (2005).

12. U.S. Food and Drug Administration, "Guidance for Industry: Questions and Answers Regarding Food Allergens, including the Food Allergen Labeling and Consumer Protection Act of 2004 (Edition 4); Final Guidance," http://www.fda.gov/Food/GuidanceComplianceRegulatoryInformation/ GuidanceDocuments/FoodLabelingNutrition/ucm059116.htm

13. Food Allergy & Anaphylaxis Network, "Advocacy, Restaurants," http:// www.foodallergy.org

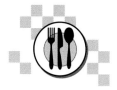

CHAPTER 3

Food Allergen Summary

Have you ever seen a breakfast menu without eggs, a lunch menu with a breadless sandwich, a dinner menu without pasta in a cream sauce, or a dessert menu without chocolate cake? I haven't and you probably haven't either. This is because these ingredients are staples of the American kitchen and key ingredients in the American diet. It would be ludicrous for a chef to even consider not having eggs, milk, cheese, bread, or fish on the menu because this is what the majority of restaurant guests expect to see on the menu.

Unfortunately for the 12 million Americans with food allergies, the top eight foods that cause allergic reactions are for the most part functional ingredients in many recipes. A chef or pastry chef cannot live without them. Ingredients such as eggs, milk, wheat, and soy and their by-products are also widely used in manufactured foods to enhance protein content and flavor, help emulsify ingredients, and to improve moisture retention. Without these ingredients, many of the foods we eat today would not be palatable.

In this chapter, we will review additional facts about these common food allergens and indentify some of the words associated with the top eight food allergens. We will also define some of the common ingredients found on food labels, describing their function in manufactured foods.

EGG: THE VERSATILE INGREDIENT

I dearly love eggs. It is hard for me not to eat an egg sandwich or omelet everyday. To a chef, eggs are as essential to cooking as air is to breathing. As Harold McGee writes in his book *On Food and Cooking: The Science and Lore of the Kitchen*:

> Eggs are one of the most versatile foods we have; they take well to a great variety of cooking techniques and combinations with other ingredients. Aside from their nutritional qualities, characteristic flavor, and yolky richness, eggs are valued for two special qualities: the ability to bind other liquids into a moist, tender solid, and the ability to form a remarkable light, delicate foam.[1]

Chefs know this quite well. The challenge in preparing traditional menu items such as pancakes, waffles, brownies, soufflés, and crème brûlée without eggs can be quite difficult or almost impossible. Guests who are allergic to eggs will avoid eggs altogether but there are some that will be looking for that adventurous chef to meet their request to recreate a rendition of one of these delicacies. There may not be a substitution for eggs in all recipes, but there are ingredients that can be used as a substitute for some.

EGG ALLERGY FACTS

- Hen's egg allergy is the second most common allergy in infancy and early childhood.
- The most allergic part of the egg is the egg white, which contains two major proteins, ovomucoid and ovalbumin.
- The incidence of egg allergy in children is about the same as milk allergy, 2% to 3%.
- Egg allergy, especially in infants with eczema, is a good predictor for other allergic diseases, as many egg-allergic infants develop additional food allergies, asthma, and hay fever.
- Egg-allergic patients who react to chicken, turkey, or game birds suffer from what is called the "chicken meat–bird egg syndrome."

- A study conducted by researchers at Hospital Sainte-Justine in Montreal, Canada, showed that out of the 60 children in the study who had been diagnosed with an egg allergy. 73% of them were able to tolerate eggs that had been cooked in a cake.[2]

IDENTIFYING EGGS ON FOOD LABELS

Figure 3.1 provides information on how to identify eggs on food labels. If you have any questions about vendor ingredient labels, always contact the vendor for additional information.

DEFINITION OF COMMON EGG
BY-PRODUCTS AND DERIVATIVES

I have been amazed by the extensive list of ingredients on some food labels with words that the average person cannot pronounce, let alone understand the meaning. When it comes to packaged foods, I wondered what function certain ingredients have on the finished product. This led me to include this information about food by-products and derivatives so you may come to better understand why manufacturers use them.

- *Albumin* is any of several water-soluble proteins that are coagulated by heat and are found in egg white, blood serum, and milk. Milk albumin is termed lactalbumin and milk albuminate, and it contains 28% to 35% protein and 38% to 52% lactose. It is used as a binder in imitation sausage, soups, and stews.[3]
- *Egg albumen* is the protein fraction of the egg, also called egg white. It makes up approximately 65% of the edible egg and is composed of approximately 87% water, 11% protein, and 1% carbohydrate. It provides a source of protein and assists foam upon whipping. It is used in meringues, cakes, and desserts.[4]
- *Egg yolk* is the yellow portion of the egg, which makes up approximately 35% of the edible egg. It is composed of 49% water, 16% protein, 32% fat, and trace carbohydrates. It is used as an emulsifier in mayonnaise, salad dressings, and cream puffs. It is also used as a source of color.[5]

EGG ALLERGEN SUMMARY

All FDA-regulated manufactured food products that contain egg as an ingredient are required by U.S. law to list the word "egg" on the product label.

Avoid foods that contain EGG or any of these ingredients:

Albumin (also spelled albumen)	Mayonnaise
Egg (dried, powdered, solids, white, yolk)	Meringue (meringue powder)
Eggnog	Ovalbumin
Lysozyme	Surimi (imitation crabmeat

EGG is sometimes found in the following:	*Keep the following in mind:*
Baked goods	
Egg substitutes	
Lecithin	Individuals with egg allergy should also avoid eggs from duck, turkey, goose, quail, etc., as these are known to be cross-reactive with chicken eggs.
Macaroni	
Marzipan	
Marshmallows	
Nougat	
Pasta	

FIGURE 3.1

HOW TO READ A LABEL FOR AN EGG-FREE DIET.

(USED WITH PERMISSION BY THE FOOD ALLERGY & ANAPHYLAXIS NETWORK, ©2010.)

MILK: THE MAIN EVENT

Like eggs, milk is a very functional ingredient in the kitchen. Milk and the foods made from milk are used to create some of the best tasting dishes. Where would we be without butter, cheese, milk, sour cream, yogurt, and ice cream? How could a chef create fabulous desserts like crème brûlée, cheesecake, and chocolate cake without milk or butter? What would a classic béchamel taste like without some rich whole milk used to make it? These are some questions that a chef could do without answering.

With the increase of food allergies to milk, there has been a rise in the use of alternative ingredients for some of these traditional items. There are now many cookbooks to choose from that omit milk from their recipes and still produce excellent tasting dishes. The vegan lifestyle, which omits any animal by-product from the diet, has also grown over the years due to different health, ethical, and economical reasons, and has prompted many chefs to create vegan options for their menus.

MILK ALLERGY FACTS

- Milk allergy is the most common childhood food allergy, affecting 2.5% of children less than age 3 and 80% of milk allergies is outgrown by age 16.[6]
- Lactoglobulin, lactalbumin and casein are three major milk proteins that are heat stable. This means that heating, or pasteurization, does not denature these proteins. These proteins are also present in other animal milk, such as buffalo, sheep, goat, camel, and ewe milk. People with milk allergies should not drink these milks.[7]
- Approximately 10% to 20% of milk-allergic children may react to beef, as cow's milk proteins are present in beef products. Some people with a milk allergy can tolerate well-done beef, as high cooking temperatures may denature the milk proteins. This may also explain why many milk-sensitive people can tolerate baked goods containing milk or egg products.[8]

IDENTIFYING MILK ON FOOD LABELS

Figure 3.2 provides information on how to identify milk on food labels. If you have any questions about ingredient labels, always contact the vendor for additional information.

MILK ALLERGEN SUMMARY

All FDA-regulated manufactured food products that contain milk as an ingredient are required by U.S. law to list the word "milk" on the product label.

Avoid foods that contain MILK or any of these ingredients:

Butter, butter fat, butter oil, butter acid, butter ester(s)	Lactulose (a synthetic sugar derived from milk)
Buttermilk	Milk (in all forms, including condensed, derivative, dry, evaporated, goat's milk and milk from animals, low-fat, malted, milk fat, nonfat, powder, protein, skimmed, solids, whole)
Casein (milk protein)	
Casein hydrolysate	
Caseinates (in all forms) (salt of casein)	
Cheese	Milk protein hydrolysate
Cottage cheese	Pudding
Cream	Recaldent®
Cheese curds	Rennet casein
Custards	Sour cream, sour cream solids
Diacetyl (a flavoring agent)	Sour milk solids
Half-and-half	Tagatose (a sweetener produced from lactose)

FIGURE 3.2
HOW TO READ A LABEL FOR A MILK-FREE DIET.
(USED WITH PERMISSION BY THE FOOD ALLERGY & ANAPHYLAXIS NETWORK, ©2010.)

MILK ALLERGEN SUMMARY (continued)	
Lactalbumin (milk protein obtained from whey), lactalbumin phosphate	Whey (in all forms; watery part of milk leftover after making cheese.)
Lactoferrin	Whey protein hydrolysate
Lacotse (milk sugar)	Yogurt
MILK is sometimes found in the following:	
Artificial butter flavor	Luncheon meat, hot dogs, sausages
Baked goods	Margarine
Caramel candies	Nisin (antibiotic substance used as a food preservative)
Chocolate	Nondairy products
Lactic acid starter culture and other bacterial cultures	Nougat

FIGURE 3.2 (CONTINUED)

DEFINITIONS OF COMMON MILK
BY-PRODUCTS AND DERIVATIVES

- *Casein* is a principal milk protein that is made from skim milk by the precipitation with lactic, hydrochloric, or sulfuric acid. It can also be produced by the use of lactic acid-producing bacteria. Caseins are usually identified according to the acid used. The principle form in which casein is used is casein salt. Rennet casein is obtained from skim milk by the precipitation with a rennet-type enzyme. Casein is used in the protein fortification of cereals, breads, and in fabricated cheeses.[9]

- *Caseinates* is the salt of casein that is produced by neutralizing the casein to pH 6.7 with calcium or sodium hydroxide. Caseinates provide a source of protein and function as emulsifiers, water binders, and whipping aids. They are used in processed meats, whipped toppings, coffee whiteners, egg substitutes, and diet foods.[10]
- *Lactalbumin* (milk albuminate) is a milk protein obtained from whey by acidifying to pH 5.2, the isoelectric point, followed by coagulation by heat. It is used for nutritional purposes as a source of protein. It is used in cereals and breads where its relative inertness minimizes complications caused by other milk proteins during baking.[11]
- *Lactic acid* is a natural organic acid present in milk, meat, and beer, but is normally associated with milk. It is heat stable, nonvolatile, and has a smooth milk acid taste. It functions as a flavor agent, preservative, and acidity adjuster in foods. It is commonly used in Spanish olives, dry egg powder, cheese spreads, and salad dressings.[12]
- *Lactose* is a disaccharide carbohydrate that occurs in mammalian milk except in whales or hippopotamuses. It is principally obtained as a cows' milk derivative. It can be termed milk sugar and consists of two sugars: glucose and galactose. It is approximately one-sixth as sweet as sugar and does not dissolve as well. It functions as a flow agent, humectant, crystallization control agent, and sweetener. It is used in baked goods for flavor, browning, and tenderizing, and in dry mixes as an anticaking agent.[13]
- *Whey* is a milk protein that remains after coagulation and removal of the curd. There are two types: sweet whey obtained during the making of rennet-type hard cheeses, such as cheddar and Swiss; and acid whey obtained during the making of acid-type cheeses, such as cottage cheese. Whey is used as a source of lactose, milk solids, and whey protein.[14]
- *Whey protein concentrate* is obtained from cheese. It is approximately 12% protein, 0.5% fat, and 65% to 70% lactose. It is use to increase the protein content of food by 33% to 55%. It also provides water control, increase in viscosity, opacity, and network interruption as a fat replacer. It is used as a fat replacer in cheese, frozen desserts, dairy products, and baked goods.[15]
- *Whey solids* are dry forms of whey. They are used as a replacement for milk solids-not-fat to provide a source or protein, solids, and flavor. It is used in baked goods, ice cream, dry mixes, and beverages.[16]

PEANUTS AND TREE NUTS ARE NOT THE SAME BUT ARE JUST AS DEADLY

Peanuts are not tree nuts but are vegetables from the legume family, which include soybeans, peas, beans, and lentils. Peanuts grow in the ground; whereas tree nuts are seeds of fruit-bearing trees.[17]

Peanut and tree nut allergies are the most serious food allergies. The use of peanuts and tree nuts in today's kitchen are included in many menu items. They can be used in breads, desserts, cookies, sauces (usually Asian), pastes, snacks, and as a topping for salads and ice cream. If you do use peanuts or tree nuts in your establishment, it is very important to know exactly where the raw product is located in the kitchen and in which recipes they are used. You should also read food labels or refer to the recipe if you are in doubt about any ingredients. The quantity of children with peanut and tree nut allergies prompted some locations at Disney to serve prepackaged peanut butter sandwiches and cookies, and eliminate peanut items from their recipes.

PEANUT AND TREE NUT ALLERGY FACTS

- More than 3 million people in the United States report being allergic to peanuts, tree nuts, or both.[18]
- Peanut allergies doubled in children from 1997 to 2002.[19]
- Peanut allergies affect 1.2% of children. Approximately 20% of children outgrow it by age 6.[20]
- Most peanut-allergic patients can safely eat other legumes such as soy or beans (95%), but they can have a concurrent allergy to tree nuts such as walnuts or pecans (25% to 50%).[21]
- Tree nut allergies (almonds, walnuts, etc.) affect 1.2% of the population.[22]
- Approximately 9% of children outgrow tree nut allergies by age 16.[23]
- Skin contact and inhalation exposure to peanut butter are unlikely to cause systemic reactions or anaphylaxis.[24]
- Anaphylaxis occurs in 20% of allergic reactions to peanuts and tree nuts.[25]

- Fatal food anaphylaxis is most often caused by peanuts (50% to 62%) and tree nuts (15% to 30%).[26]
- One peanut contains about 200 mg of protein. Very trace amounts, as little as 2 mg of protein, or 1/250th of an average peanut, can trigger an allergic reaction.[27]

DOES LIVING IN DIFFERENT COUNTRIES AFFECT FOOD ALLERGIES?

There is a higher rate of peanut allergy in Chinese-Americans than in the Mainland China population. Differences in sensitization rates in the United States and China could be explained by consumption of roasted peanuts in the United States, whereas in China and other Asian countries, peanuts are consumed boiled or fried.[28]

DOES FOOD PROCESSING CHANGE PROTEINS

Thermal processing (a high temperature, sterilization process used by manufacturers to increase canned goods stability) may enhance certain foods' allergenic potential by changing their susceptibility to digestion, altering their allergen structure, or destroying the allergen.[29]

IDENTIFYING PEANUTS ON FOOD LABELS

Figure 3.3 provides information on how to identify peanuts on food labels. If you have any questions about ingredient labels, always contact the vendor for additional information.

IDENTIFYING TREE NUTS ON FOOD LABELS

Figure 3.4 provides information on how to identify tree nuts on food labels. If you have any questions about ingredient labels, always contact the vendor for additional information.

PEANUT ALLERGEN SUMMARY

All FDA-regulated manufactured food products that contain peanut as an ingredient are required by U.S. law to list the word "peanut" on the product label.

Avoid foods that contain PEANUTS or any of these ingredients:

Artificial nuts	Monkey nuts
Beer nuts	Nut meat
Cold pressed, expeller pressed, or extruded peanut oil	Nut pieces
Goobers	Peanut butter
Ground nuts	Peanut flour
Mixed nuts	Peanut protein hydrolysate

PEANUT is sometimes found in the following:

African, Asian (Chinese, Indian, Indonesian, Japanese, Thai, and Vietnamese), and Mexican dishes	Enchilada sauce
Baked goods, breakfast cereals, and cereal bars	Marzipan
Candy, confectionery, and savory snacks	Mole sauce
Chili	Nougat
Egg rolls	

FIGURE 3.3

HOW TO READ A LABEL FOR A PEANUT-FREE DIET.

(USED WITH PERMISSION BY THE FOOD ALLERGY & ANAPHYLAXIS NETWORK, ©2010.)

PEANUT ALLERGEN SUMMARY (continued)	
Keep the following in mind:	
Mandelonas are peanuts soaked in almond flavoring.	A study showed that unlike other legumes, there is a strong possibility of cross-reaction between peanuts and lupine.
The FDA exempts highly refined peanut oil from being labeled as an allergen. Studies show that most allergic individuals can safely eat peanut oil that has been highly refined (not cold pressed, expeller pressed, or extruded peanut oil).	Arachis oil is peanut oil.
	Many experts advise patients allergic to peanuts to avoid tree nuts as well.
	Sunflower seeds are often produced on equipment shared with peanuts.

FIGURE 3.3 (CONTINUED)

TREE NUT ALLERGEN SUMMARY	
All FDA-regulated manufactured food products that contain a tree nut as an ingredient are required by U.S. law to list the specific tree nut on the product label.	
Avoid foods that contain NUTS or any of these ingredients:	
Almonds	Nangai nuts
Artificial nuts	Natural nut extract (e.g., almond, walnut)
Beechnut	Nut butters (e.g., cashew butter)
Brazil nuts	nut meal
Butternut	Nut paste (e.g., almond paste)
Cashews	Nut pieces
Chestnuts	Nutmeat
Chinquapin	Pecans
Coconut	Pesto
Filberts/hazelnuts	Pili nut
Gianduja (a chocolate-nut mixture)	Pine nuts (also referred to as Indian, pigñolia, pignolia, piñon, and pinyon nuts)
Ginkgo nut	Pistachios

FIGURE 3.4

HOW TO READ A LABEL FOR A TREE NUT-FREE DIET.

(USED WITH PERMISSION BY THE FOOD ALLERGY & ANAPHYLAXIS NETWORK, ©2010.)

TREE NUT ALLERGEN SUMMARY (continued)	
Hickory nuts	Praline
Litchi/lichee/lychee nut	Shea nut
Macadamia nuts	Walnuts
Marzipan/almond paste	
TREE NUTS are sometimes found in the following:	
Black walnut hull extract (flavoring)	Nut oils (e.g., walnut oil, almond oil)
Natural nut extract	Walnut hull extract (flavoring)
Nut distillates/alcoholic extracts	
Keep the following in mind:	
Mortadella may contain pistachios.	
There is no evidence that coconut oil and shea nut oil/butter are allergenic.	
Many experts advise patients allergic to tree nuts to avoid peanuts as well.	

FIGURE 3.4 (CONTINUED)

FISH AND SHELLFISH

Fish and shellfish are common foods on many menus and are an important part of the healthy diet. According to the National Marine Fisheries Service, it is estimated that Americans eat 16.3 pounds of seafood each year, which is actually far less than doctors' recommend. It is pretty easy to substitute or even eliminate seafood from a menu item to make it safe for a guest with a seafood allergy. The major concern with a seafood allergy is the chance of cross-contact with cooking equipment, utensils, and hidden ingredients in a menu item.

FISH AND SHELLFISH ALLERGY FACTS

- An estimated 2.3% of Americans—that's nearly 7 million people—are allergic to seafood, including fish and shellfish.
- Salmon, tuna, and halibut are the most common kinds of fish to which people are allergic. Shrimp, crab, and lobster cause the most shellfish allergies.
- Allergy to fish and shellfish is considered lifelong; once a person develops the allergy, it is unlikely that they will outgrow it.
- Approximately 40% of those with a fish allergy first experienced an allergic reaction as an adult.
- Approximately 60% of those with a shellfish allergy first experienced an allergic reaction as an adult.
- To avoid a reaction, strict avoidance of seafood and seafood products are essential. Always read ingredient labels to identify fish and shellfish ingredients. In addition, avoid touching fish and shellfish, going to the fish market, and being in an area where shellfish are being cooked (the protein in the steam may present a risk).[30]

IDENTIFYING FISH ON FOOD LABELS

Figure 3.5 provides information on how to identify fish on food labels. If you have any questions about ingredient labels, always contact the vendor for additional information.

FISH ALLERGEN SUMMARY	
Since products made with fish or fish ingredients are easy to identify, it is relatively easy to identify on ingredient labels.	
FISH are divided into two categories: Flat and Round	
Anchovies	Pike
Bonito	Plaice
Cod	Salmon
Eel	Sardine
Flounder	Shark
Grouper	Snapper
Haddock	Sole
Hake	Swordfish
Halibut	Trout
Mackerel	Tuna
Foods that may contain FISH	
Caesar salad contains anchovies in either the salad or dressing	Hot dogs, bologna, and ham may contain fish flavoring
Caviar is fish eggs	Pizza toppings may contain anchovies
Roe is unfertilized fish eggs	Worcestershire sauce contains anchovies
Marinara sauce may contain anchovies	

FIGURE 3.5

FISH ALLERGEN SUMMARY.

(FROM T.E.A.C.H.: FOOD ALLERGEN TRAINING MANUAL, ALLERGY CHEFS, INC., ©2010.)

SHELLFISH ALLERGEN SUMMARY

All FDA-regulated manufactured food products that contain crustacean shellfish as an ingredient are required by U.S. law to list the specific crustacean shellfish on the product label.

Avoid foods that contain SHELLFISH or any of these ingredients:	*SHELLFISH are sometimes found in the following:*
Barnacle	Bouillabaisse
Crab	Cuttlefish ink
Crawfish (crayfish, ecrevisse)	Fish stock
Krill	Glucosamine
Lobster (langouste, langoustine, scampo, coral, tomalley)	Seafood flavoring (e.g., crab or clam extract)
Prawns	Surimi (imitation crab)
Shrimp	

Mollusks are not considered major allergens under food labeling laws and may not be fully disclosed on a product label.

Doctors may advise their patients to avoid mollusks or these ingredients:	
Abalone	Periwinkle
Clams (cherrystone, geoduck, littleneck, pismo, quahog)	Scallops

FIGURE 3.6

HOW TO READ A LABEL FOR A SHELLFISH-FREE DIET.

(USED WITH PERMISSION BY THE FOOD ALLERGY & ANAPHYLAXIS NETWORK, ©2010.)

SHELLFISH ALLERGEN SUMMARY (continued)	
Cockle	Sea cucumbers
Cuttlefish	Sea urchin
Limpet (lapas, opihi)	Snails (escargot)
Mussels	Squid (calamari)
Octopus	Whelk (turban shell)
Oysters	

FIGURE 3.6 (CONTINUED)

IDENTIFYING SHELLFISH ON FOOD LABELS

Figure 3.6 provides information on how to identify shellfish on food labels. If you have any questions about ingredient labels, always contact the vendor for additional information.

SOY: THE MANUFACTURERS' INGREDIENT

The soybean is one of the most important legumes in the world. It is one of the least expensive proteins to produce and is high in protein and magnesium, and is a good source of dietary fiber and omega-3 fatty acids. Studies have shown that there are many health benefits like lowering cholesterol and reducing the risk of heart disease.

The reason it is so widely used in manufacturing is because the bean contains 40% protein and 18% oil, and the protein contains all the essential amino acids. This makes it an inexpensive protein replacement in processed foods. The bean can be processed into soybean flour, protein concentrate, protein isolate, and soybean oil.[31] Since soy protein is so widely used in manufacturing, it limits the amount of processed foods people with a soy allergy can eat. So reading food labels to identify soy ingredient is very important when serving a guest with a soy allergy.

SOY ALLERGY FACTS

- Soybean allergy is less common than cow milk allergy in infants and children, about 3 in every 1000.[32]
- Symptoms of soy allergy are typically mild, although anaphylaxis is possible.
- Soybean allergy is one of the more common food allergies, especially among babies and children.[33]
- Unlike other food reactions, except for wheat, the onset of a soybean reaction may be delayed several hours.[34]
- The U.S. Food and Drug Administration exempts highly refined soybean oil from being labeled as an allergen.[35]

IDENTIFYING SOY ON FOOD LABELS

Figure 3.7 provides information on how to identify soy on food labels. If you have any questions about ingredient labels, always contact the vendor for additional information.

DEFINITIONS OF COMMON SOY
BY-PRODUCTS AND DERIVATIVES

- *Lecithin* is an emulsifier that is now commercially obtained from soybeans but used to be obtained from egg yolks. It is used in margarines as an emulsifier and anti-spatter agent; in chocolate to control flow properties by reducing viscosity and reducing the cocoa butter content 3% to 5%; as a wetting agent in cocoa powder, fillings, and beverage powders; as an antisticking agent in griddling fat; and in baked goods to assist the shortening mix with other dough ingredients and to stabilize air cells.[36]

ALWAYS CHECK WITH YOUR GUEST

Most individuals allergic to soy can safely eat soy lecithin but it is always good to double check with the guest with the soy allergy before serving any items with soy lecithin.

- *Soybean flour* is made from defatted soybean, having a protein content in excess of 50%. It is used in doughnuts, cereal, bread, and sausage products for protein fortification and binding.[38]
- *Soybean oil* is obtained from the seed of the soybean legume. It is made up of 86% unsaturated fatty acids with linoleic and oleic being the two main fatty acids. It can be either hydrogenated or nonhydrogenated, and is used in shortenings and margarine in the hydrogenated form, and in salad dressings and cooking oils as nonhydrogenated.[39]

ARE HIGHLY REFINED OILS SAFE?

Studies show most allergic individuals can safely eat soy and peanut oil that has been highly refined (not cold pressed, expeller pressed, or extruded soybean oil).[37] Oils that have not been highly refined still contain an intact protein molecule so are not recommended for consumption by a food allergic guest.

- *Soybean protein* is most commonly prepared as soybean flour (50% protein), soybean concentrate (70% protein), and soybean protein isolate (90% protein). It can be used in sausages, snack foods, and meat analogs to provide emulsification, binding, moisture and texture control, and protein fortification.[40]
- *Textured vegetable protein* (TVP) is a vegetable protein that is processed and extruded to form beeflike strips, meatlike nuggets, or other analogs. In the dehydrated form, the analogs are crunchy and upon hydration become moist and chewy. Soy protein is the most popular protein source, but other vegetable proteins include peanut and wheat. It is also called textured soy flour or textured soy protein.[41]

SOY ALLERGEN SUMMARY	
All FDA-regulated manufactured food products that contain soy as an ingredient are required by U.S. law to list the word "soy" on the product label.	
Avoid foods that contain SOY or any of these ingredients:	
Edamame	Soya
Miso	Soybeans (curd and granules)
Natto	Soy protein (concentrate, hydrolyzed isolate)
Shoyu	Soy sauce
Soy (soy albumin, soy cheese, soy fiber, soy grits, soy ice cream, soy milk, soy nuts, soy sprouts, soy yogurt)	Tamari
	Tempeh
	Textured vegetable protein (TVP)
	Tofu
SOY is sometimes found in the following:	
Asian cuisine	Vegetable gum
Vegetable broth	Vegetable starch

FIGURE 3.7

HOW TO READ A LABEL FOR A SOY-FREE DIET.

(USED WITH PERMISSION BY THE FOOD ALLERGY & ANAPHYLAXIS NETWORK, ©2010.)

WHEAT: PART OF EVERY MENU

Wheat is a staple of the American diet and can be seen on every menu and grocery store shelf in the form of sandwiches, croutons, breaded items, crackers, pasta, cakes, cookies, desserts, and even beer. It has been cultivated for at least 6,000 years and is the world's largest cereal-grass crop. Its status as a staple is second only to rice. The reason it is so popular is that, unlike other cereals, wheat contains a high level of gluten, a protein that provides elasticity to baked goods.[42]

A wheat allergy is different from celiac disease. Whereas a wheat allergy is an immunoglobulin E (IgE)-mediated response to the wheat protein, celiac disease is a permanent adverse reaction to gluten. Those with celiac disease will not lose their sensitivity to this substance.[43] Even though there is a difference between the two, you should handle them with the same precautions.

WHEAT ALLERGY FACTS

- A wheat allergy is primarily common in children and is usually outgrown before they reach adulthood.[44]
- People with a wheat allergy have an IgE-mediated response to wheat protein and may tolerate other grains.[45]
- Symptoms of wheat allergy reaction can range from mild to severe.

IDENTIFYING WHEAT ON FOOD LABELS

Figure 3.8 provides information on how to identify wheat on food labels. If you have any questions about ingredient labels, always contact the vendor for additional information.

DEFINITIONS OF COMMON WHEAT BY-PRODUCTS AND DERIVATIVES

- *Hydrolyzed vegetable protein (HVP)* is a flavor enhancer obtained from vegetable proteins such as wheat gluten, corn gluten, defatted soy flour, and defatted cottonseed. Once the protein is hydrolyzed it is a refined liquid that consists of amino acids, monosodium glutamate, amino acid derivatives, salt, and water. It is used to improve flavors in soups, dressings, meats, snack foods, and crackers.[46]

- *Wheat gluten* is a water-soluble complex protein fraction separated from wheat flour. It is also called gum gluten in its fresh extracted wet form. In its dry form, it can absorb two to three times its weight in water. It is used in baked goods because it has the ability to form adhesive, cohesive masses, films, and three-dimensional networks. Gluten formation imparts dough strength, gas retention, structure, water absorption, and retention with breads, cakes, and other baked goods. It is also used as a formulation aid, binder, filler, and tableting aid.[47]

- *Wheat starch* is the starch obtained from wheat. It produces a lower viscosity and more tender gels than starch obtained from corn or sorghum. It has a gelatinization range about 10°C lower than corn or waxy maze starch. It is used in the baking industry to permit the use of hard wheat flour in baked goods and it functions as a binder in breading and batter goods.[48]

WHEAT ALLERGEN SUMMARY

All FDA-regulated manufactured food products that contain wheat as an ingredient are required by U.S. law to list the word "wheat" on the product label. The law defines any species in the genus *Triticum* as wheat.

Avoid foods that contain WHEAT or any of these ingredients:

Bread crumbs	Matzoh, matzoh meal (also spelled matzo, matzah, or matza)
Bulgur	Pasta
Cereal extract	Seitan
Club wheat	Semolina
Couscous	Spelt
Cracker meal	Sprouted wheat
Durum	Triticale
Einkorn	Vital wheat gluten
Emmer	Wheat (bran, durum, germ, gluten, grass, malt, sprouts, starch)
Farina	Wheat bran hydrolysate

FIGURE 3.8

HOW TO READ A LABEL FOR A WHEAT-FREE DIET.

(USED WITH PERMISSION BY THE FOOD ALLERGY & ANAPHYLAXIS NETWORK, ©2010.)

WHEAT ALLERGEN SUMMARY (continued)	
Flour (all purpose, bread, cake, durum, enriched, graham, high gluten, high protein, instant, pastry, self-rising, soft wheat, steel ground, stone ground, whole wheat)	Wheat germ oil
	Wheat grass
	Wheat protein isolate
Hydrolyzed wheat protein	Whole wheat berries
Kamut	
WHEAT *is sometimes found in the following:*	
Glucose syrup	Starch (gelatinized starch, modified starch, modified food starch, vegetable starch)
Soy sauce	Surimi (imitation crabmeat)

FIGURE 3.8 (CONTINUED)

CORN: IS IT AN ALLERGY OR INTOLERANCE?

There has been some controversy over whether corn causes an allergic reaction or is merely a food intolerance. If you ask someone that has had a severe reaction to corn and corn derivatives, they would tell you it was an allergy. There have been a few documented cases of corn-induced asthma and rhinitis, but it is quite rare to find a corn-induced food allergy. The reason I am including corn is because I have served many guests with corn allergies/intolerances over the past several years. It can be very challenging to prepare food for a guest with a corn allergy/intolerance because corn derivatives are in many foods. You may not encounter many people with a corn allergy/intolerance but when you do, make sure to read food labels carefully to ensure that a corn ingredient is not present.[*]

CORN IS IN ALMOST EVERY PROCESSED FOOD

Corn is a grain that was first grown and cultivated over 5,600 years ago by the Aztec tribes in Mexico. It is now one of the most abundant grains grown throughout the world and is planted on 70 to 80 million acres of land in the United States. We can enjoy it fresh, frozen, or canned. Fresh corn on the cob is available year round, peaking in flavor in the summer months. It is as sweet as sugar and wonderful to eat boiled, steamed, or grilled. Manufacturers love it too because it can be made into corn bran, flour, and gluten; cornmeal; oil; starch; sugar (dextrose); syrup; syrup solids; and vinegar. These derivatives are an inexpensive substitute used to add flavor, sweetness, protein, and binding in many manufactured foods.

IDENTIFYING CORN ON FOOD LABELS

Figure 3.9 provides information on how to identify corn on food labels. If you have any questions about ingredient labels, always contact the vendor for additional information.

---

[*] Since corn is not recognized by the FDA as a top food allergen, it does not have to be listed in the ingredient statement as its common name. If there is a question concerning an ingredient, show the label to the guest so they can make the final decision.

CORN ALLERGEN SUMMARY
Avoid foods that contain CORN or any of these ingredients:
Corn (bran, flour, meal, starch)
Corn gluten
Corn sugar (dextrose)
Corn syrup, high fructose corn syrup, and corn syrup solids
Maize
Grits
Hominy
Corn oil
Glucose

CORN is sometimes found in the following:	
Baked goods/cooking ingredients	Cream pies
Baking mixes for biscuits, doughnuts, pancakes, and pies	Glucose products
Baking powder	Graham crackers
Batters and deep-frying mixtures	Oleo or margarine
Bleached wheat flour	Powdered sugar
Breads and pastries	Tortillas
Cakes	Vanilla extract
Cereals	Vinegar (distilled)
Cookies	Xanthan gum

FIGURE 3.9

CORN ALLERGY/INTOLERANCE SUMMARY.

(FROM T.E.A.C.H.: FOOD ALLERGEN TRAINING MANUAL, ALLERGY CHEFS, INC., ©2010.)

CHAPTER REVIEW

The major food allergens are in many ways an essential part of today's menus and manufactured goods and are used to create an array of different types of foods. Even with the enactment of the Food Allergen Labeling and Consumer Protection Act, manufacturers have not shied away from using milk, egg, soy, and wheat ingredients in their processed foods. Even with the labeling law, it is still important to read food labels and look for consumer advisory statements. Many food allergen ingredients can be in foods that you might not think would contain them; therefore, reading food labels is an essential part to ensuring you can identify hidden food allergens in manufactured foods.

ENDNOTES

1. Harold McGee, *On Food and Cooking: The Science and Lore of the Kitchen* (New York: Scribner, 1984), 54.
2. Paul J. Hannaway, MD, *On the Nature of Food Allergy* (Marblehead, MA: Lighthouse Press, 2007), 82–83.
3. Robert S. Igoe and Y. H. Hui, *Dictionary of Food Ingredients,* 4th ed. (Gaithersburg, MD: Aspen Publishers, Inc., 2001), 5.
4. Ibid., 51.
5. Ibid., 52.
6. Hugh A. Sampson and Scott H. Sicherer, "Food Allergy," *Journal of Allergy Clinical Immunology* 117 (2006): S470–S475.
7. Hannaway, 78.
8. Ibid.
9. Igoe and Hui, 32.
10. Ibid., 32.
11. Ibid., 81.
12. Ibid.
13. Ibid., 82.
14. Ibid., 153.
15. Ibid., 154.
16. Ibid.
17. Hannaway, 91.
18. Ann Munoz-Furlong, Hugh A. Sampson, and Scott H. Sicherer, "Prevalence of Self-Reported Seafood Allergy in the U.S" [abstract], *Journal of Allergy and Clinical Immunology* 113 suppl (2004): S100.

19. Scott H. Sicherer et al. "Prevalence of Peanut And Tree Nut Allergy in the United States Determined by Means of a Random Digit Dial Telephone Survey: A 5-Year Follow-Up Study," *Journal of Allergy and Clinical Immunology* 112 (2003):1203–1207.
20. Hugh A. Sampson and Scott H. Sicherer, "Peanut Allergy: Emerging Concepts and Approaches for an Apparent Epidemic," *Journal of Allergy and Clinical Immunology* 120 (2007): 491–503.
21. Ibid.
22. American Academy of Allergy, Asthma, and Immunology (AAAAI), "Allergy Statistics," http://www.aaaai.org/media/statistics/allergy-statistics.asp
23. Ibid.
24. S. J. Simonte et al. "Relevance of Casual Contact with Peanut Butter in Children with Peanut Allergy," *Journal of Allergy and Clinical Immunology* 112 (2003): 180–182.
25. Scott H. Sicherer et al. "Clinical Features of Acute Allergic Reactions to Peanut and Tree Nuts in Children," *Pediatrics* 102, no. 1 (1998): e6.
26. Corinne A. Keet, MD, and Robert A. Wood, MD, "Food Allergy and Anaphylaxis," *Immunology Allergy Clinic of North America* 27 (2007): 193–212.
27. Hannaway, 91.
28. Ibid.
29. Ibid.
30. Food Allergy & Anaphylaxis Network (FAAN), "Common Food Allergens," http://www.foodallergy.org/section/common-food-allergens1
31. Igoe and Hui, 135.
32. Hannaway, 99.
33. Food Allergy & Anaphylaxis Network (FAAN), "How to Read a Label for a Soy-Free Diet," 2008.
34. Hannaway, 100.
35. FAAN, "How to Read a Label for a Soy-Free Diet," 2008.
36. Igoe and Hui, 83.
37. FAAN, "How to Read a Label for a Soy-Free Diet," 2008.
38. Igoe and Hui, 135.
39. Ibid.
40. Ibid.
41. Ibid., 144.
42. Sharon T. Herbst and Ron Herbst, *The New Food Lover's Companion*, 3rd ed. (New York: Barron's Educational Series, Inc.), 736.
43. Food Allergy & Anaphylaxis Network (FAAN), "Wheat Allergy," http://www.foodallergy.org/
44. Ibid.
45. Ibid.
46. Igoe and Hui, 73.
47. Ibid., 153.
48. Ibid.

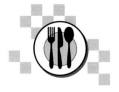

CHAPTER 4

Special Diets

Food allergies are very serious and require the elimination of specific foods, but it is not the only special dietary request you may encounter in your restaurant. There are many people on special diets due to an illness, disease, or food intolerance, and others may have some belief or lifestyle choice that makes them follow a "preference" diet. Autism, celiac disease, diabetes, lactose intolerance, and phenylketonuria (PKU), which are related to a disease or food intolerance, were the most common special diets I encountered while working at Disney. These diets have to be managed by the elimination or avoidance of certain foods. The most common preference diets were vegetarian and vegan. People following preference diets do so for personal, religious, or ethical reasons.

According to a global research report conducted by AllergyFree Passport, there are over 117 million North Americans managing a special diet. This represents a significant number of potential customers who are probably not eating at your restaurant because their options are limited or the staff is not properly trained to manage their requests.

WHAT IS FOOD INTOLERANCE?

Food intolerance is any adverse reaction to food that is not caused by the immune system. This kind of reaction may sometimes be called "delayed food allergy" by certain medical experts. Symptoms are not the same for all individuals and side effects may be delayed for several hours after eating. Delayed reactions make it difficult to diagnose food intolerances. Elimination diets and special tests can be conducted to identify the offending food or foods. Symptoms can include gastrointestinal distress, headaches, sinus and breathing problems, and chronic fatigue. Food intolerances are not life threatening, but it is still important to handle these dietary requests the same way you would a food allergy. For more information on food intolerances, refer to *The Complete Guide to Food Allergy and Intolerance,* 4th ed., by Jonathan Bronstoff and Linda Gamlin.

AUTISM

You may not have met someone that has autism let alone cooked for a family with an autistic child and may be wondering why I have included autism in this book. I think it is important to make food service professionals aware of this growing disorder in America.

In the past several years, I have encountered many families with autistic children that required special diets. Many of them needed gluten-free and casein-free foods or wanted certain types or brands of food prepared for their child. Many of these requests were easy to accommodate because the food was readily available in our kitchen.

In 2009, I was asked by the American Culinary Federation to conduct several seminars on special diets that related to childhood diseases such as autism, diabetes, obesity, and food allergies. During the presentations, I learned that some of the participants had an autistic child, knew of a family with an autistic child, or had served families with autistic children. They were very interested in learning more. What also encouraged me to include this information about autism was the growing number of companies that support autism research and the foods they manufactured to meet the requirements for autistic children.

WHAT IS AUTISM?

According to the National Institute of Neurological Disorders and Stroke, autism spectrum disorder (ASD) is a range of complex neuro-development disorders, characterized by social impairments; communication difficulties; and restricted, repetitive, and stereotyped patterns of behavior. Autistic disorder, sometimes called autism or classical ASD, is the most severe form of ASD. Other conditions along the spectrum include a milder form known as Asperger syndrome, the rare condition called Rett syndrome, and childhood disintegrative disorder and pervasive developmental disorder not otherwise specified (PDDNOS). Although ASD varies in character and severity, it occurs in all ethnic and socioeconomic groups, affecting every age group.[1]

AUTISM FACTS

- One out of 6 children is diagnosed with a developmental disorder and/or behavioral problem.
- One in 166 children is diagnosed with an autism spectrum disorder.
- Males are four times more likely to have autism spectrum disorder than females.

There is no cure for ASD, but there are a variety of treatments that can are designed to remedy specific symptoms and can bring about substantial improvements. Educational and behavioral interventions and medications may help and can be prescribed by a doctor, but there are a number of controversial therapies or interventions that are available to people with ASD. Most of these are not supported by scientific studies but are supported by parents and some doctors because they have seen actual results.[2]

For some time now, food intolerance and sensitivities have been receiving more attention as possible causes for autistic behavior. Researchers have recently detected the presence of abnormal levels of peptides (amino acids) in the urine of autistic individuals. It is thought that these peptides may be due to the body's inability to break down certain proteins into amino acids. It is also thought that these proteins, once absorbed into the brain, act as a drug that dramatically changes a child's behavior.

SENSORY ISSUES TO FOOD

I have talked to many parents that have explained to me that their autistic child has issues with flavors or textures of certain foods in their mouths. Their child will only eat specific brands of food because it is familiar to them.

These proteins are gluten found in wheat, barley, and rye, and casein found in dairy products like milk, cheese, and yogurt. Many parents who have removed these foods from their child's diet have seen dramatic, positive changes in their child's health and behavior.

SPECIAL DIETS FOR AUTISM

The gluten-free casein-free (GFCF) diet and the specific carbohydrate diet (SCD) are two diets used to help reduce the symptoms of autism. Whereas the GFCF diet eliminates all gluten and dairy products, the SCD allows some dairy products but eliminates lactose (milk sugar). SCD is also very strict in what foods are allowed. Certain meats, fish, eggs, vegetables, whole grains, nuts, and low-sugar fruits make up the diet. The goal of the SCD is to restore the health of the digestive system so it can absorb nutrients for overall health. Refer to Figure 4.1 for a casein-free diet guide.

WHAT YOU SHOULD KNOW ABOUT
SERVING AN AUTISTIC CHILD

In the event that you are requested to prepare a meal for an autistic child remember these steps:

- Prepare the food as directed by the parent or family member.
- Adhere to specific brands of food if requested (i.e., Dannon yogurt vs. Yoplait yogurt).
- If a GFCF diet is requested, follow all food allergen safety procedures so that the food will not be contaminated by gluten or casein.

In most situations the family will contact you ahead of time to find out if you can accommodate their child's dietary request. If you are unable to accommodate them, they may still come in bringing premade food for their child. For more information about autism contact ANDI, Autism Network for Dietary Intervention, at P.O. Box 335 Pennington, NJ 08534-0335 or visit its Web site at www.autismndi.com.

CELIAC DISEASE

Of the many dietary requests I have seen over the years, guests looking for gluten-free meals have been the most common. This is supported not only by the fact that 1 in 100 Americans have celiac disease, there are many companies producing gluten-free foods that are offered in local grocery stores, and books and magazines dedicated to this subject now cover whole shelves at bookstores. If you consider serving any guests with special diets, this is the one to focus on.

Celiac disease, also called celiac sprue or gluten-sensitive enteropathy, is a digestive disease that damages the small intestine and interferes with absorption of nutrients from food. People with celiac disease cannot tolerate gluten, a protein found in wheat, rye, and barley. Gluten is found mainly in foods but may also be found in everyday products such as medicines, vitamins, nutritional supplements, and lip balm.[3]

When people with celiac disease eat foods or use products containing gluten, their immune system responds by damaging or destroying the villi (tiny, fingerlike protrusions lining the small intestines). Villi normally allow nutrients from food to be absorbed through the walls of the small intestine into the bloodstream. This is how the body stays healthy. Without healthy villi, a person will become malnourished, regardless of how much they eat.[4]

Celiac disease is genetic and often runs in family members. Sometimes the disease occurs after surgery, pregnancy, childbirth, viral infection, or severe emotional stress.

Casein-Free Diet Guide	
Foods That Contain Casein	**Casein-Free Alternatives**
Milk	Rice, soy or potato-based milks
Cream	Pareve creams and creamers
Half & Half	Mocha mix
Yogurt	Rice, soy or coconut milk yogurts
Sour cream	Tofutti Brand Sour Cream®
Cheese (most, except some soy based)	Tofutti brand Better Than Cream Cheese®
Butter	Earth Balance Natural Buttery Spreads
Sherbet	Sorbet
White or milk chocolate	Dark chocolate
Ice cream	Soy, rice and coconut-based frozen desserts (not all flavors)
Ice milk	Italian ices
Creamed soups and soup bases	Imagine Brand Soups and Swiss Chalet Specialty soup bases

FIGURE 4.1

CASEIN-FREE DIET GUIDE.

(REPRINTED WITH PERMISSION FROM LIVING WITHOUT MAGAZINE, ©2010 BELVOIR MEDIA GROUP. FOR MORE INFORMATION GO TO WWW.LIVINGWITHOUT.COM.)

Casein-Free Diet Guide (continued)	
Foods That Contain Casein	**Casein-Free Alternatives**
Puddings and custards	Ecocuisine soy puddings
Whey	Coconut butter and milk
All bovine milk and milk products contain casein. Avoid foods derived from goat and sheep milk, as well as cow dairy products.	Kosher pareve foods are casein-free. Foods certified as kosher nondairy or pareve are free of dairy proteins.
Foods That May Contain Casein	
Margarine	Semi-sweet chocolate
Tuna fish	Hot dogs
Dairy-free cheese (most brands)	Lunch meats
Lactic acid	Sausage
Artificial flavorings	Ghee
Dairy-Free May Contain Casein	
Many nondairy foods contain casein proteins. Avoid foods that contain an ingredient with casein or caseinate.	

FIGURE 4.1 (CONTINUED)

FACTS AND STATISTICS

- There are approximately 1 in 100 to 1 in 200 people worldwide that have celiac disease.
- There are approximately 1 in 100 Americans with celiac disease, which is at least 3 million Americans.
- Ninety-seven percent of people remain undiagnosed.[5]
- Among people who have a first-degree relative—a parent, sibling, or child—diagnosed with celiac disease, as many as 1 in 22 people may have the disease.
- A high prevalence of celiac disease is also found in people with type 1 diabetes, thyroid disease, Down syndrome and other disorders.
- Eating even a small amount of gluten can damage the small intestines.
- Hidden sources of gluten include additives such as modified food starch, preservatives, and stabilizers made from wheat.[6]

SYMPTOMS

Symptoms of celiac disease vary from person to person and occur in the digestive system or in other parts of the body. Digestive symptoms are more common in infants and young children, whereas adults are less likely to have digestive symptoms. Adults typically can have other symptoms that make it difficult to diagnose celiac disease because the same symptoms can be found in other diseases like irritable bowel syndrome (IBS), iron-deficiency anemia caused by menstrual blood loss, inflammatory bowel disease, diverticulitis, intestinal infections, and chronic fatigue syndrome.[7]

- Symptoms in infants and young children: bloating, gas, diarrhea, weight loss, poor growth, irritability, dental enamel abnormalities, and anemia
- Symptoms for older children and adults vary from mild to severe: anemia, nausea, bloating, gas, diarrhea or constipation (or both), lactose intolerance, weight loss, mouth ulcers, extreme fatigue, bone and joint pain, easy bruising of the skin, menstrual irregularities, miscarriage, infertility in women and men, migraines, depression, and elevated liver enzymes[8]

If left untreated, celiac disease can result in nutritional deficiencies, increased risk of osteoporosis, intestinal cancers, neurological disorders, reproductive complications, and development of other autoimmune diseases. The only treatment for celiac disease is a strict gluten-free diet for life.

GLUTEN DEFINED

Gluten is the common name for proteins (prolamins) found in wheat, rye, and barley. The specific names of the toxin proteins are gliadin in wheat, secalin in rye, and hordein in barley. All forms of wheat, rye, and barley must be strictly avoided.[9] (See Figure 4.2 and Figure 4.3.)

There are many foods that are naturally gluten-free including plain meats, poultry, fish, eggs, legumes, nuts, seeds, milk, yogurt, cheese, fruits, and vegetables. There are also many gluten-free grains and flours that taste great and are readily available (Figure 4.4).

Distilled alcoholic beverages and wine are also allowed, but beers made with barley are off limits. If you enjoy a good beer now and then, you are in luck. Today there are a variety of gluten-free beers on the market. Even before Anheuser-Busch came out with a gluten-free beer called Redbridge, we were receiving requests for a gluten-free beer from our guests with celiac disease. Once we started offering it in our restaurants, guests sent thank you letters for providing this simple pleasure. Today, you can find many restaurants and bars offering gluten-free beer

DISTILLED SPIRITS, VINEGAR, AND VANILLA

In the past, there has been confusion about the safety of alcoholic beverages, vinegar, and vanilla by the gluten-free community. After a careful review by *Gluten-Free Living* magazine of the distillation process, it was found that the gluten peptides couldn't survive the distillation process, which renders the product safe. This is only true for products that are distilled, which beer is not, and malt vinegar because malt is added back in after the distillation process. (For more detailed information concerning this subject see *Gluten-Free Living* magazine, Sept./Oct. and Nov./Dec. 1999 and vol. 8, no. 3, 2003.)

Ale	Lager
Atta*	Malt
Barley (flakes, flour, pearl)	Malt extract, syrup, and flavoring
Beer	Malt vinegar
Brewer's yeast	Malted milk
Bulgur	Matzoh, matzoh meal
Couscous	Modified wheat starch
Dinkel (also known as spelt)**	Rye
Durum**	Seitan****
Einkorn**	Semolina
Emmer**	Spelt (also known as farro or faro; dinkel)
Farina	Triticale
Farro or faro (also known as spelt)**	Wheat
Fu***	Wheat bran
Graham flour	Wheat flour

FIGURE 4.2

FOOD AND INGREDIENTS CONTAINING GLUTEN. (REPRINTED FROM GLUTEN-FREE DIET: A COMPREHENSIVE RESOURCE GUIDE BY SHELLEY CASE, RD. ©2010 CASE NUTRITION CONSULTING INC.)

Hydrolyzed wheat protein	Wheat germ
Kamut**	Wheat starch

*   Fine whole-meal flour made from low-gluten, soft-textured wheat used to make Indian flatbread (also known as chapatti flour).

**   Types of wheat.

*** A dried gluten product derived from wheat that is sold as thin sheets or thick, round cakes. Used as a protein supplement in Asian dishes such as soups and vegetables.

**** A meat-like food derived from wheat gluten used in many vegetarian dishes. Sometimes called "wheat meat."

FIGURE 4.2 (CONTINUED)

because they see the value of offering an alternative for the many people suffering from celiac disease. Following are additional gluten-free beers you may want to try:

- Bards' Tale by Bard's Tale Beer Company
- New Grist by Lake Front Brewery
- Greens' Gluten Free Beers by St. Peter's Brewery
- Nick Stafford's Hambleton Ales

ARE OATS SAFE TO EAT?

Oats were once considered off limits for people with celiac disease or gluten sensitivity but after 12 years of research conducted in Europe and the United States, it was revealed that the moderate consumption of oats is safe for a majority of children and adults. Children can safely consume ¼ to ½ cup and adults can consume ½ to ¾ cup of dry rolled oats. The studies used pure, uncontaminated oats, but it should be noted that a very small number of individuals might not even tolerate pure oats.[10]

The problem with commercial oats is that these products are contaminated with wheat, barley, or rye, which occurs during harvesting, transportation, storage, milling, processing, and packaging. The good news is that there are companies in the United States, Canada, and Europe that

Baking and cooking sprays
Breads and other baked goods
Breading, coating mixes, and panko
Broths
Cake frostings and icings
Cereals
Croutons
Curry paste
Imitation bacon and seafood (surimi)
Oats (Commercial oats may be contaminated during growing, harvesting, processing, and packaging. Only purchase oats that are guaranteed gluten-free.)
Pastas
Soups such as cream, chowder, and bisques
Sauces such as béchamel, veloutés, and espagnole (brown sauce) and reductions
Specially prepared mustards
Soy sauce (which is often made from wheat and soy)

FIGURE 4.3

POSSIBLE SOURCES OF GLUTEN.

(ADAPTED FROM GLUTEN-FREE DIET: A COMPREHENSIVE RESOURCE GUIDE BY SHELLEY CASE, RD. ©2010 CASE NUTRITION CONSULTING INC.)

Seasonings
Salad dressings and marinades
Snack foods
Stuffing and dressings
Prepared meats (e.g., deli meats, hot dogs, hamburger patties, imitation seafood)
Flavored coffees and teas
Some candies (e.g., licorice) and chocolate bars
Soup and sauce thickeners (roux)
Worcestershire sauce

FIGURE 4.3 (CONTINUED)

produce pure, uncontaminated specialty oats. Here in the United States, gluten-free oats can be found on many health food or specialty grocery store shelves. Following is a list of the North American companies:

- Bob's Red Mill, www.bobsredmill.com
- Cream Hill Estates (Lara's brand), www.creamhillestates.com
- Avena Foods (Only Oats™), www.onlyoats.com
- Gifts of Nature, www.giftsofnature.net
- Gluten-Free Oats, www.glutenfreeoats.com
- Montana Gluten-Free Processers, www.montanaglutenfree.com

GLUTEN-FREE LABELING

The last several years have seen an increase in the use of "gluten-free" labeling on a variety of foods, including raw, cooked, and baked foods. This was spurred by the boost in sales of gluten-free products on the

Amaranth	Potato starch
Arrowroot	Quinoa
Buckwheat	Rice (black, brown, glutinous/sweet, white, wild)
Corn	Rice bran
Flax	Rice polish
Indian ricegrass (Montina™)	Sago
Legume flours (bean, chickpea/garbanzo, lentil, pea)	Sorghum
Mesquite flour	Soy
Millet	Sweet potato flour
Nut flours (almond, hazelnut, pecan)	Tapioca (cassava/manioc)
Potato flour	Teff

FIGURE 4.4

GLUTEN-FREE FLOURS, CEREALS, AND STARCHES.

(ADAPTED FROM GLUTEN-FREE DIET: A COMPREHENSIVE RESOURCE GUIDE BY SHELLEY CASE, RD. ©2010 CASE NUTRITION CONSULTING INC.)

market, which was estimated at $1.6 billion in retail sales ending in 2008 and is estimated to grow to $2.2 billion in sales by 2012. Since the Food and Drug Administration (FDA) has not yet defined the term *gluten-free*, many consumers are frustrated and confused about which products are truly safe to eat. Food manufactures would also like to have a gluten-free labeling standard. This would eliminate uncertainty or misunderstanding regarding labeling and limit the use of the term gluten-free to truly gluten-free foods. With a standard in place, it would make all manufacturers adhere to the same labeling requirements.

Ever since the creation of the Food Allergen Labeling and Consumer Protection Act, the FDA was directed by Congress to define the term gluten-free to comply with a statutory mandate. The FDA was to issue a proposed rule that would define and permit the use of the term gluten-free on the labeling of foods no later than two years after the law's enactment date (August 2006), and a final rule by no later than four years after the law's enactment date (August 2008).

The FDA proposes that the definition of gluten-free to mean a food bearing this claim in its labeling does not contain any one of the following:

- An ingredient that is a prohibited grain
- An ingredient that is derived from a prohibited grain and that has not been processed to remove gluten
- An ingredient that is derived from a prohibited grain and that has been processed to remove gluten, if the use of that ingredient results in the presence of 20 parts per million (ppm) or more gluten in the food

The FDA is also proposing to define the term gluten-free for voluntary use in the labeling of foods. Once a final federal decision is made, manufacturers who wish to label their products as gluten-free may do so, but only if the food bearing the label meets the proposed regulatory guidelines. The FDA has proposed synonyms for the gluten-free labeling claim to include "free of gluten," "without gluten," and "no gluten."[11]

Shelley Case, RD, recently published the most current information on the gluten-free labeling law in the latest edition of Gluten-Free Diet: A Comprehensive Resource Guide. She writes, "(FDA) will be publishing a final rule to define the food labeling term "gluten-free" sometime after it solicits and considers the public comments it receives on the agency's safety assessment report on gluten exposure in individuals who have celiac disease. FDA's intent to conduct this safety assessment was mentioned in the preamble of the proposed rule. A Federal Register notice will be published to announce the availability of FDA's draft safety assessment report. Because of this intermediate step, it is premature to estimate when the final rule will be published. However, interested individuals may wish to periodically check FDA's website for updates on the safety assessment report and the final rule."

WHAT IS THE DIFFERENCE
BEWEEN HVP AND HPP

According to Ann Whelan in *Gluten-Free Living* magazine, for the ingredients hydrolyzed vegetable protein (HVP) or hydrolyzed plant protein (HPP) on labels: "The source of the protein should always be listed on the label of a food that contains HVP or HPP. If it is 'hydrolyzed soy protein,' it would be gluten free; if it is 'hydrolyzed wheat protein' it would not be gluten free."

GLUTEN-FREE CERTIFICATION
PROGRAM FOR RESTAURANTS

There are a number of associations that offer certification programs for restaurants that has proven to increase business for these establishments. If you are interested in learning more about these programs please contact the following groups.

- The Gluten-Free Restaurant Awareness Program™ (GFRAP). Gluten Intolerance Group of North America®, 31214 124 Ave SE, Auburn, WA 98092; e-mail: GFRAP@comcast.net; Web site: www.GlutenFreeRestaurants.org; phone: 253-833-6655.
- GREAT Kitchens offered by National Foundation for Celiac Awareness. Web site, www.CeliacCentral.org/great; phone: 215-325-1306, ext. 300.

WHAT YOU SHOULD KNOW ABOUT SERVING
PEOPLE WITH CELIAC DISEASE

Since there are a variety of gluten-free foods that can be prepared for the main entrée, having items available to replace bread, breakfast pastries, and desserts should be considered. Having these items in your restaurant will make a significant difference in the overall dining experience for your guests. Premade gluten-free breads, pastries, and desserts can be purchased online or from health food stores and many of them can be kept in the freezer and retrieved when requested. A list of products and manufacturers can be found in Chapter 8. For more information about the gluten-free diet, including foods/ingredients allowed and to avoid; gluten-free labeling; meal planning; recipes; cross-contamination issues; a detailed listing of gluten-free products and manufacturers; and other helpful resources see *Gluten-Free Diet: A Comprehensive Resource Guide* by Shelley Case, RD, at www.glutenfreediet.ca.

DIABETES

Diabetes is a growing epidemic in America. With the increase in obesity in all ages, diabetes has become more prevalent, especially in children and teenagers. Most of this is due to unhealthy eating habits coupled with a lack of exercise.

According to the U.S. Department of Health and Human Services, diabetes is a group of diseases marked by high levels of blood glucose resulting from defects in insulin production, insulin action, or both. Diabetes can lead to serious complications and premature death, but people with diabetes can take steps to control the disease and lower the risk of complications.

FACTS AND STATISTICS

- Diabetes occurs when the body does not produce or properly use insulin, which is a hormone that helps the body process sugar.
- There are two major types of diabetes:
  - Type 1 diabetes was previously called insulin dependent (no insulin produced) or juvenile-onset diabetes. This develops when the body's immune system destroys pancreatic beta cells, the only cells in the body that make hormone insulin that regulates blood glucose. People with type 1 diabetes must take insulin daily to manage this disease. This form of diabetes usually affects children and young adults, but may occur at any age. In adults, type 1 diabetes accounts for 5% to 10% of all diagnosed cases of diabetes. Risk factors may be autoimmune, genetic, or environmental.

- Type 2 diabetes was previously called noninsulin dependent (body is insulin resistant or deficient) or adult-onset diabetes. In adults, type 2 diabetes accounts for about 90% to 95% of all diagnosed cases of diabetes. It usually begins as insulin resistance, a disorder in which the cells do not use insulin properly. As the need for insulin rises, the pancreas gradually loses its ability to produce it. Type 2 diabetes is associated with older age, obesity, family history of diabetes, history of gestational diabetes (a form of glucose intolerance diagnosed during pregnancy), impaired glucose metabolism, physical inactivity, and race/ethnicity.
- Diabetes can lead to serious complications, such as blindness, kidney damage, cardiovascular disease, and lower-limb amputations, but people can lower the occurrence of these and other diabetes complications by controlling blood glucose, blood pressure, and blood lipids (fats).
- Prevalence of diagnosed and undiagnosed diabetes in the United States, all ages, 2007
  - Total: 23.6 million people or 7.8% of the population have diabetes
  - Diagnosed: 17.9 million people
  - Undiagnosed: 5.7 million people
- Diabetes can be managed by monitoring blood sugar levels, eating foods that are low in carbohydrates; counting carbohydrates, calories, and dietary fiber; managing portion size; and daily exercise.[12]

WHAT YOU SHOULD KNOW ABOUT SERVING PEOPLE WITH DIABETES

Many people with diabetes can manage their own diet without asking for nutritional information but there are some diabetics that will ask. What may add to the increase in the questions concerning the nutritional content of restaurant menu items is the passing of the Patient Protection and Affordable Care Act. On March 23, 2010, President Barack Obama signed this act into law. Part of the act consists of Section 4205 that requires restaurants with 20 or more locations nationally to add calorie counts to menus, menu boards, and drive-through menu boards for standard menu items. It also requires covered restaurants to make additional nutritional data available upon request.[13]

The additional nutritional data will be required to be in writing, on the premises, and include the following:

- Calories
- Calories from fat
- Total fat
- Saturated fat
- Cholesterol
- Sodium
- Carbohydrates
- Sugars
- Dietary fiber
- Protein

This will make it easier for restaurants that fit this category to answer customer nutritional questions, but what about the restaurants that do not have to offer this information? By law, you are not required to provide this information to the customer if asked. If you are asked about nutritional information and do not have a reliable source or a way to provide this information, it is best not to share any information. People with diabetes require accurate information to manage their insulin intake.

If you want to better serve your customers with diabetes, here are some helpful tips:

- Chefs can call their local hospital dietitian or check the American Dietetics Association Web site to find a registered dietitian.
- Purchase the book *The CalorieKing®: Calorie, Fat, & Carbohydrate Counter*, 20th Anniversary Edition. This book provides basic nutritional information on common foods and similar restaurant menu items. I have suggested this book to many guests seeking nutritional information on restaurant foods. I have also used it to provide guests with some general carbohydrate data for standard restaurant menu items.
- Show the guest the package label that will contain the nutritional information.
- If a guest asks you to prepare their meal with specific portion sizes, follow their request. It is easy to portion out their meal using a scale or portioning utensils.

REAL LIFE EXPERIENCE

My dad has been diabetic for more than 40 years and he has done a great job managing his diabetes through monitoring his blood sugar, appropriate insulin intake, diet, and exercise. The biggest challenge he has had was getting restaurants to portion his food appropriately and getting a great tasting sugar-free dessert.

IS IT REALLY SUGAR-FREE?

The Food and Drug Administration has established guidelines for the labeling of foods that claim to be sugar-free. If you plan on serving sugar-free options it is important that the menu item is correctly labeled.

- *Unsweetened* means that no compound with a sweet taste has been added to a food or drink.
- *Without added sugar, No added sugar,* and *No sugar added* mean that the product does not contain any sugar, either natural or substitute.
- *Sugar-free* means that a food has less than 0.5 grams of sugar per serving.
- *Reduced sugar* means there is at least a 25% reduction of sugar from the original product.

- Offer a sugar-free dessert. This is the part of the meal that most diabetics skip. Most desserts are too high in sugar and the alternative they are frequently offered is fresh fruit. If I were the guest, I would be thinking, "When I am out for dinner, I want to have a great tasting dessert, not just fruit. I can get that at home." Here is your opportunity to provide a tasty dessert and increase revenue.
- Work with a local vendor or bakery to have them prepare a sugar-free dessert that you can keep on hand.

Making an effort to provide information or portion meals to meet this request will create loyal guests that will return to your establishment.

LACTOSE INTOLERANCE

You may not receive many guest requests for specially prepared meals because they are lactose intolerant, but since many digestive diseases require people to avoid milk and milk products, it is important to understand a little more about it.

Lactose intolerance is the inability or insufficient ability to digest lactose, a sugar found in milk and milk products. The body produces the enzyme lactase that breaks down lactose in the small intestine. When the body does not produce enough or no longer produces the lactase enzyme the body can no longer digest the sugar and certain symptoms occur.[14]

People sometimes confuse lactose intolerance with a cow's milk allergy but these are two different problems. Milk allergy most commonly appears in the first year of life, whereas lactose intolerance occurs more often in adulthood.

Primary lactase deficiency develops over time and begins at about age 2 when the body begins to produce less lactase. Most children who have lactase deficiency do not experience symptoms until late adolescence or adulthood. Secondary lactase deficiency results from injury to the small intestine that occurs with severe diarrheal illness, celiac disease, Crohn's disease, or chemotherapy. This type of lactase deficiency can occur at any age but is most common in infancy.[15]

There are approximately 30 to 50 million Americans adults with lactose intolerance. The pattern of primary lactose intolerance appears to have a genetic component, and is commonly found in certain ethnic groups:

- 95% of Asians
- 60–80% of African Americans and Ashkenazi Jews
- 80–100% of American Indians
- 50–80% of Hispanics

Lactose intolerance is least common among northern Europeans, who have a lactose intolerance prevalence of only 2%.[16]

Symptoms

People with lactose intolerance may feel symptoms 30 minutes to 2 hours after consuming a food that contained milk or milk products. Symptoms range from mild to severe, based on the amount of lactose consumed and the amount a person can tolerate. Common symptoms include:

- Abdominal pain
- Abdominal bloating
- Gas
- Diarrhea
- Nausea

What You Should Know about Serving People with Lactose Intolerance

Many people with lactose intolerance will avoid milk products all together. Others will take the lactase enzyme pill before a meal to help them digest the lactose, or order a vegetarian or vegan meal to keep the symptoms from occurring. With a significant number of Americans with lactose intolerance, it is a good idea to have alternative products available, such as lactose-free milk, soy or rice milk, and nondairy creamers, along with an assortment of nondairy desserts.

PHENYLKETONURIA (PKU)

What Is PKU?

According to the National Institute of Child Health and Human Development, PKU is an inherited disorder of metabolism that can cause intellectual and developmental disabilities (IDD) if not treated. In PKU, the body cannot process a portion of the protein called phenylalanine (Phe), which is in almost all foods. If the child's Phe level in the blood is too high, the brain can become damaged. A person with PKU cannot eat more than .05 grams of protein per meal.

REAL LIFE EXPERIENCE

The first guest I served with phenylketonuria was a 5-year-old boy. His family was coming to Disney for the first time, and their son had never eaten a meal in a restaurant. When I spoke with the mother about his dietary requirements, I could not believe what I heard. He could not eat any type of protein like chicken, beef, pork, turkey, eggs, milk, beans, and the list went on. He was on a special formula to supply all of his protein needs and had a very limited diet as you can imagine. She provided me with a list of foods and products from a company called Cambrooke Foods that specialized in low-protein foods. I could understand a person being allergic to a food, but when I found out that there were people that could not digest proteins, any kind of proteins, I was shocked.

We made arrangements to have the food shipped in and distributed to their dining locations with specific instructions on food preparation and service. We were fortunate that the guest notified us ahead of time because it took two weeks to receive the products and it was not cheap. I could not believe how expensive the products were since they did not contain protein. Come to find out, the formulation and processing of the products was time consuming, which added to the costs. Even though there were some issues with acquiring the products and getting it to each location, the chefs did a great job making this family's dining experiences "magical."

Now that there was a new special diet to learn about, I ordered a variety of Cambrooke products to conduct my own product evaluations. I was truly amazed at the quality and taste of the products. The best products were the macaroni and cheese; portobello spinach ravioli; and Camburgers, a mixture of chopped portobello mushroom and vegetables. Upon completion of the tests, we added eight low-protein products that covered breakfast, lunch, and dinner.

Phenylalanine is found in the following foods:

- Meat, fish, poultry
- Milk, eggs, cheese
- Ice cream
- Legumes and nuts
- Flour
- Aspartame, which can be found in Diet Coke and other diet products

Foods that can be eaten include:

- Fruits
- Vegetables
- Low-protein breads, pastas, and cereals

Symptoms

All babies born in the U.S. hospital are now tested for PKU within 48 hours of birth. This is to make it easier to diagnose and treat them early. Children that go untested may appear normal at birth but by 3 to 6 months will begin to lose interest in their surroundings. By one year of age, they may be underdeveloped and have less skin pigmentation than other children. If left undiagnosed they may develop severe IDD.

What You Should Know about Serving People with PKU

If you get a request from a guest with PKU it is important that you follow their instructions carefully. They may simply ask you for some fruits and vegetables, since they may have brought their own food to eat. If your company policy allows you to prepare food that a guest brings with them, make sure that it is an unopened package, follow the directions, and use all food allergen safety guidelines that will be described later in this book.

PREFERENCE DIETS

Preference diets can be more than a request for vegetarian or vegan menu items. It could also include ingredient substitutions, removal of ingredients from a plate or menu item, or simply a request for an item that is not on the menu. Some guests may make this type of request and disguise it as a food allergy or intolerance when it may only be a "food aversion" as described in Chapter 1. Regardless of how the request is made, in today's challenging economy where restaurants are battling for every consumer dollar, it is vital that a restaurant do what it can to meet every request.

AN OVERVIEW OF VEGETARIANISM

Vegetarianism is one of the most common preference diets you will encounter in the restaurant business. During the last several years at Disney, there was an increase in requests for vegetarian meals. This encouraged us to add a vegetarian offering to every menu. Even with having a vegetarian item on every menu, many of the guests wanted more than just a basic salad, soup, or pasta primavera with cheese. They were demanding something new and exciting. I believe the demand for more creative and tasty vegetarian dishes was fueled by the growth of organic food markets, countless books on the benefits of living a vegetarian diet and Food Network chefs demonstrating how great tasting vegetarian food can be. This has influenced people not following the vegetarian diet to buy vegetarian meals.

VEGETARIAN STATISTICS

According to a study conducted by *Vegetarian Times*, 3.2% of U.S. adults, or 7.3 million, follow a vegetarian-based diet. Of this number, 0.5%, or 1 million, follow a vegan diet. In addition, 10% of U.S. adults, or 22.8 million people, say they try to follow a vegetarian-inclined diet.[17]

VEGETARIANISM DEFINED

Vegetarianism is the practice of living on plant-based foods, with or without the use of eggs or dairy products, but excluding entirely the consumption of any part of an animal, including chicken, fish, or seafood.

TYPES OF VEGETARIANS

There are many types of vegetarians that may be contradictory to the definition but the person may still consider himself or herself a vegetarian.

- Lacto (milk) is a vegetarian who does not eat meat, poultry, fish, or eggs but will eat dairy products.
- Ovolacto (*ovo* means "egg" in Portuguese) is a vegetarian who does not eat meat, poultry, and fish but will eat eggs and dairy products.
- Pesco is a vegetarian that will eat fish.
- Pollo is a vegetarian that will eat chicken.
- Flexitarian, semi-, or demi- is a vegetarian that frequently chooses to avoid meats.
- Fruitarians exclude all foods of animal origin as well as pulses (the dried seeds of some legumes) and cereals. Their diet mainly consists of raw and dried fruits, nuts, honey, and olive oil.

VEGAN

The vegan diet has more restrictions than the vegetarian diet. Vegans exclude all foods of animal origin. Their diet consists of fruits, vegetables, vegetable oils, cereals, pulses such as beans and lentils, nuts, and seeds. This diet is not as unexciting as it may sound due to the wide variety of meat alternatives, soy-based yogurts and frozen desserts, biscuits, chocolates, milks, and so forth available that are completely free of any animal products. Most vegans also exclude animal products from their lifestyle (e.g., wool, leather, soaps that contain animal fats, and products tested on animals).

RAW CUISINE

Raw cuisine is based on uncooked organic foods. Food cannot be heated above 118°F because vital enzymes that aid digestion will be destroyed. The diet consists of fruits, vegetables, nuts, seeds, and oils. It is believed that a diet of living fruits and vegetables add vitality to a person's health and render them virtually disease-free.

REASONS FOR BECOMING VEGETARIAN OR VEGAN

- Religious—It is written in the Book of Genesis, "Then God said, 'I give you every seed-bearing plant on the face of the whole earth and every tree that has fruit with seed in it. They will be yours for food'" (Genesis 1:29).
  - Other religions that live the vegetarian lifestyle are Brahmanism, Buddhism, Jainism, Zoroastrianism, Seventh Day Adventists, and The Order of the Cross.
- Hunter-gatherers theory—Kalahari Bushmen and the Australian aborigines are hunter-gatherers and the proportion of plant-based foods to animal-based foods in their total diet is approximately 81% to 19%.
- Nutritional—Eating foods associated with these diets has healthy benefits like reducing fat and cholesterol.
- Ethical—Cruelty to animals and more efficient use of the world food resources has driven people to avoid animal products.
- Economic—Nonmeat products are, on the average, less expensive.

WHY OFFER VEGAN OPTIONS

As obesity in America continues to rise, the government will be asking Americans to reduce their portion size and eat healthier. This will hopefully encourage more people to try and lead a healthier lifestyle. Those that choose to make the change will still be going out to eat and will expect the food service industry to meet their needs.

Creating vegan meals can be a little challenging, but it can be beneficial to your operation to offer at least one vegan option. Here are a several reasons to add a vegan option to your menu.

- Lower cost of ingredients can keep food cost down
- Saves the server or chef time discussing options with the guest because a vegan option will already be on the menu
- Vegan options
    - Cover vegetarian requests
    - Cover vegan requests
- Cover requests for meals that are milk- and egg-free

WHAT YOU SHOULD KNOW ABOUT SERVING PEOPLE ON A VEGETARIAN OR VEGAN DIET

These lifestyle diets are easy to accommodate. Here are some simple tips to provide more vegetarian or vegan options on your menu.

- Be flexible in modifying menu options
- Offer sauces prepared with vegetable stock instead of beef or chicken stock
- Offer a vegan soup daily
- Prepare croutons from bread that is vegan and use oil instead of butter to coat the bread
- Prepare a vegan dessert or offer vegan sorbet or a nondairy, vegan frozen dessert

THE BEST VEGETARIAN/VEGAN BURGER

The veggie burger is the most common vegetarian/vegan option on today's menus and many of them are not good. The worst thing for a vegetarian or vegan diner to eat is a bad veggie burger. The best one I have eaten is the Malibu Burger made by Gardenburger®. It is a vegan veggie-style burger made from a blend of organic whole grains (brown rice and rolled oats) and organic vegetables (corn, carrots, onions, green peppers) seasoned with organic spices. It is available in a 3.2 ounce/48 count case from many food service distributors.

CHAPTER REVIEW

The bottom line for food service operations is to stay competitive in today's market. You need to stay current with the lifestyle diet trends. More people will be making decisions that will affect their diet, health, and pocketbook. Many of these decisions will affect where they choose to eat.

Your next steps should be to properly train your team on how to handle food allergy and special dietary requests, how to serve food safely, and enhance your menu with a variety of options that are easy to execute. This will position your operation ahead of the competition and place you in good standing with the community.

ENDNOTES

1. National Institute of Neurological Disorders and Stroke (NINDS), "Autism Fact Sheet," http://www.ninds.nih.gov/disorders/autism/detail_autism.htm, 2010.
2. NINDS, "Autism Fact Sheet."
3. National Digestive Diseases Information Clearinghouse (NDDIC), "Celiac Disease," NIH Publication No. 08-4269 September 2008, 1, http://www.digestive.niddk.nih.gov/ddiseases/pubs/celiac/
4. NDDIC, "Celiac Disease," 1.
5. Shelley Case, BSc, RD, "Celiac Disease & the Gluten-Free Diet," May 2010, 20. http://www.glutenfreediet.ca/img/Celiac.pdf (accessed December 2010).
6. NDDIC, "Celiac Disease," 6.
7. Ibid., 2.
8. Case, 1.
9. Ibid., 2.
10. Ibid., 2.
11. U.S. Food and Drug Administration, "Questions and Answers on the Gluten-Free Labeling Proposed Rule," http://www.fda.gov/Food/Labeling-Nutrition/FoodAllergensLabeling/GuidanceComplianceRegulatory-Information/ucm111487.htm
12. Department of Health and Human Services, Centers of Disease Control and Prevention, "National Diabetes Fact Sheet," 2007, http://www.cdc.gov/diabetes/pubs/pdf/ndfs_2007.pdf

13. National Restaurant Association, "Q&A: New Federal Nutrition-Disclosure Rules for Certain Restaurants," April 7, 2010, http://www.restaurant.org/pdfs/advocacy/menulabeling_faq.pdf

14. National Digestive Diseases Information Clearinghouse (NDDIC), "Lactose Intolerance," NIH Publication No. 09-2751, June 2009, 1, http://digestive.niddk.nih.gov/ddiseases/pubs/lactoseintolerance/

15. NDDIC, "Lactose Intolerance," 1.

16. National Institute of Child Health and Human Department, "Lactose Intolerance: Information for Health Care Providers," NIH Publication No. 05-5305B, January 2006, 2.

17. Vegetarian Times, "Vegetarianism in America," http://www.vegetariantimes.com/features/archive_of_editorial/667

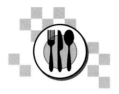

PART II

Skills

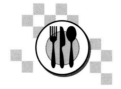

THE REAL LIFE EXPERIENCES OF GINA CLOWES, MOM AND PRESIDENT OF ALLERGYMOMS.COM

As I was writing this book I kept thinking to myself, how am I going to really get you, the reader, to understand how challenging, serious, and rewarding serving people with food allergies can be? I can describe my experiences and explain processes and procedures that will help you develop a sound food allergen safety program, but how will you really get it? I thought it was important to talk to the people who live with food allergies everyday. That is why I reached out to a few friends and colleagues and asked them to share their real life experiences with you.

Throughout the following chapters, Gina Clowes, founder and director of AllergyMoms.com, will be sharing her experiences with her son's food allergies and restaurants. Clowes takes food allergies so seriously that she became a certified life coach, specializing in helping parents with children who have food allergies. I hope her experiences will convey how important food allergen safety is and why it is so important to become educated and trained in this field.

The Reality of Restaurant Dining with Food Allergies

After a few mishaps in restaurants after my son was first diagnosed with multiple food allergies, I learned that restaurants were no longer a safe place for us. I had to learn to cook allergy-friendly meals, and I would do it often. There are many other challenges that we continue to deal with. One of the most difficult parts of managing a food allergy is traveling. When you're on the road, you almost have to eat some meals on the go.

We eat at only one local restaurant and did not do so until my son was six years old. His name is Daniel and he is allergic to milk, eggs, peanuts, tree nuts, wheat, and sesame. When I approached the restaurant, it was very interested and motivated to serve allergic customers. I had to do a little more investigating, which included me reading over many of the restaurant's recipes and working out a system with them that worked for both of us. With some work and partnership, we have it down to a science. We treasure our times at this restaurant (Mad Mex, Cranberry Township, Pennsylvania location) and visit there at least twice a month. Outside of our local area, the restaurants at Disney (Walt Disney World® and Disneyland®) are the only places we've found consistency in their ability to handle multiple food allergies.

Gina Clowes

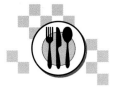

CHAPTER 5

Getting Started

The following chapters will describe the steps that you can take to develop your own food allergy program. These chapters will cover building a communication process, service and kitchen management training tips, and menu and recipe creation with appropriate ingredient substitutions and packaged products that will help you create your own menu offerings. Before I go on, I want to say one thing: *If you are not 100% sure you want to start a food allergy program, don't!* You and your staff have to take all food allergy requests seriously and understand what your responsibilities are in order for the program to be successful. There is no maybe, sort of, or I think we can do this. Guests with food allergies will be putting their trust in you and your team that they will be eating a safe meal. So you have to get it right every time.

BUILDING A COMMUNICATION PROCESS

In my role as Culinary Development and Special Dietary Needs Manager for Walt Disney World Resort, my task was to develop the food allergy and special diets policies and procedures for over 450 food and beverage locations. That included the following styles of service:

- Outdoor kiosks
- Quick service restaurants
- Food courts/fast casual restaurants
- Family buffet and table service restaurants
- Fine dining
- Catering

This seemed like a daunting task but Disney is known for its exceptional service and people that can make anything happen. I was fortunate to work with talented cast members who helped me develop a successful dietary program. To make any program work, it was essential to build a communication process first.

Building a communication process is a very important part in developing a successful food allergy program. Why? Because you need to ensure that everyone in your food service operation is properly informed of your policies and procedures. It is equally important to inform the guest what you can do to accommodate their request. You do not want one of your team members to communicate the wrong information from a guest to the kitchen or visa versa.

Webster's Dictionary defines *communication* as "the imparting or exchanging of information and news; a letter or message containing such information or news; the successful conveying or sharing of ideas and feelings, or a means of connecting between people or places." Each of these definitions has a very important meaning and the following processes utilize these definitions in their development. Here are the steps that can help you develop a successful communication process:

- Designate a person to lead the process
- Organize a communication team
- Develop and implement communication forms
- Develop easy to understand communication message points
- Continue to monitor feedback from operations and guests

DESIGNATE A PERSON TO LEAD THE PROCESS

Regardless of the size of your company or food service operation, designating one person to lead the process is very important. For the sake of this book, we will call this person the special diets manager (SDM). The SDM's responsibilities should include but not be limited to the following:

- Being the contact person for your team members
- Assisting team members with answering guest questions
- Conducting research
- Controlling internal and external communication
- Product development
- Training

In selecting this person, it is important to consider his or her background. The SDM should have actual restaurant experience and understand how the front of the house (FOH) and back of the house (BOH) operate since this is where the food allergy request is handled.

The first step for the SDM is to put together a committee made up of the following team members: administrative personnel (i.e., administrative assistant), receiver or food procurement specialist, head or lead server, FOH manager, BOH manager or chef, training specialist, food safety specialist, and a legal consultant (Figure 5.1).

Each team member's experience can provide valuable information about current food allergy and special dietary requests and the challenges being faced by both FOH and BOH team members. Collecting, analyzing, and prioritizing this information is also important. The number and types of dietary requests will help you decide what type of training is necessary, what foods are needed to meet these requests, and how to develop the proper communication messages for your guests and staff.

WHAT EACH TEAM MEMBER BRINGS TO THE TABLE

Each team member has specific knowledge, skills, and abilities in their job that will help in the development of appropriate message points and procedures. By involving your team members from the beginning, you will have a better chance of getting their buy-in to any changes due to implementing a food allergy program.

Special Diets Committee

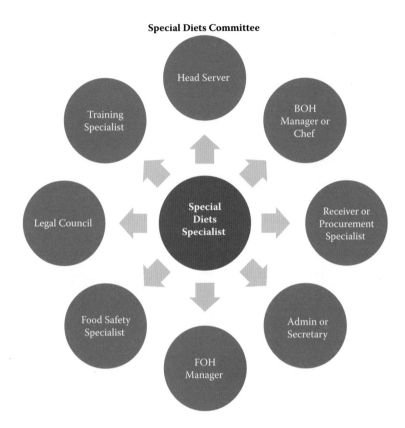

FIGURE 5.1
SPECIAL DIETS COMMITTEE.

- *Administrative support* provides communication with guests in verbal and written form, and supports the creation of internal and external documents.
- *Receiver or food procurement specialists* provide the knowledge of proper food handling and can assist in acquiring special dietary products. This will be discussed further in Chapter 7, "Kitchen Management."
- *Head or lead servers* provide the skills of daily service operation and have an insight of how servers may view new policies. This helps in the development of important message points to this audience. This group is critical in the overall success of your food allergy program. Many food allergy reactions come from servers relaying incorrect or incomplete information to the kitchen or improper food handling on their part.

- *Front-of-the-house managers* provide the knowledge of FOH operations and are a key part in relaying information to the kitchen.
- *Back-of-the-house managers or chef* is the most important person in this process. He or she provides the knowledge, skills, and abilities of kitchen operations, recipe ingredients, and preparation techniques and will ultimately be responsible for the preparation of the food.
- *Food safety specialists* provide the knowledge of current government food safety and food allergy policies (if any exist in your state) and can support leadership in training and implementation of the food allergy program.
- *Legal consultants* will provide the legal support and can review all written documents when necessary.

PUTTING TOGETHER A COMMUNICATION TEAM

This may sound redundant because you may have thought that you already put together a communications team. That was a committee to collect information to help develop your communication plan. Depending on the size of your operation, you may use some of the operations team for your communications team but you will need to divide the duties.

The communications team should consist of administrative support team members that have time to answer phone calls, read e-mails, and relay information between the guest and the operators. If you do not have sufficient administrative support, this may be the responsibility of the special diets manager, a front-of-the-house manager, or chef. I would suggest against the latter in a large operation because it can be overwhelming for one person to handle this part along with running an operation.

RESPONSIBILITIES

The communications team should be responsible for the following:

- Writing policies and procedures
- Communicating information to your guests and team members

- Updating contact and Web site information, and recipe or ingredient statements
- Tracking guest communications and information

It is best to have only a few people controlling the internal and external information so that it stays consistent. There are times when a guest will call back and talk to a different team member and get contradicting information, which could lead to a disappointed guest or, worse, a sick guest.

PREPARING COMMUNICATION DOCUMENTS

In today's society, there are so many ways to communicate with our guests. Phones, e-mail, Internet, Facebook, Twitter, and blogs are easily accessible to most people. Unfortunately, you have little control over many of these avenues of communication. What can be controlled is the written content in your documents and Web site. Verbal communication is not as effective as written communication since many people only hear what they want to hear. I have learned this from talking to guests with food allergies.

Having your policies and procedures in writing with the ability to share them with your guests for review prior to their dining experience can save time and eliminate confusion and misunderstandings. Be advised that anything in writing can be used in a court of law, so have your documents reviewed by a legal consultant.

TYPES OF DOCUMENTS

The following are examples of written documents that can be used to share information with your guests prior to their dining experience. Since these ideas were created for a multiunit operation with lodging accommodations, some may not apply to you.

- *The dietary request information letter* should include general information about your operation such as a phone number or e-mail address of the department or person handling the requests, types of food allergy and dietary requests you are willing to accommodate, your basic food allergy procedures, and frequently asked questions (Figure 5.2).

Welcome to JJ's Seafood Bar & Grill,

Thank you for contacting us about your special dietary request ahead of time. This will help us communicate the correct information between you and our service and kitchen staff to make your dining experience exceptional.

The service staff, chefs, and managers at JJ's Seafood Bar & Grill take all food allergy and special dietary requests seriously. We have spent extensive time training our staff on the appropriate service and cooking procedures to reduce that chance of cross-contact occurring with any special dietary meal prepared.

Because of the diversity of our menu items and cooking procedures, we only handle the following dietary requests:

- Celiac disease and gluten sensitivities
- Lactose intolerance
- Food allergies
  - Milk
  - Egg
  - Peanut
  - Tree nut
- Vegetarian
- Vegan

We offer specialty breads, pastas, and desserts that are free of gluten, milk, eggs, peanuts, and tree nuts that are prepared in our "Food Allergen Safety Zone" or by a brand-name company that specializes in dietary products.

For more information, please contact our Special Diets Department at XXX-XXX-XXXX between the hours of 8 a.m. to 5 p.m. EST, Monday–Friday or e-mail us at jjspecialdiets@comcast.net.

Frequently Asked Questions: Please visit our Web site and click on the FAQ tab on the bottom of the home screen.

FIGURE 5.2
DIETARY REQUEST INFORMATION LETTER.

LEGAL DISCLAIMER

Following is an example of a legal disclaimer that should appear on your documents:

> Our company has used reasonable efforts to prevent the introduction of the allergen of concern into the food through close attention during our sourcing, preparation, and handling processes. However, please be advised that you have to use your own individual discretion on making an informed decision based on the information we have provided you. Our company cannot guarantee that allergens may not have been introduced during another stage of the food chain process, or even inadvertently, by us.

- *Product information sheet(s)* should include basic information about general products and their ingredients and where they are available, if in a multiunit location such as a theme park, cruise ship, or hotel (Figure 5.3).
- *The dietary data sheet* should contain guest information such as name and age (age is important when it comes to the types of food that can be suggested to the guest), day and evening phone numbers, e-mail address, date of visit, guest allergy, and types of food the guest can eat (see Figure 5.4 and Figure 5.5).
  - The guest should fill out this form so the information is input correctly. If one of your team members fills out the form, the guest should review it before it is sent to the restaurant.
- *A food allergen notebook* is a pocket-sized notebook that can be used by the server, manager, and chef or person in charge to document any discussion with the food allergic guest (Figure 5.6). It should contain areas to write the guest's table number, date, and time the discussion took place; servers', manager's, or chef's name; the top eight food allergens; and an area to write the type of food being prepared for the guest. We will talk about this notebook more in Chapters 6 and 7.

These documents are helpful in reducing guest anxiety, minimizing guest questions when they arrive at your restaurant, informing your team members of current company policies, and keeping documentation of a guest's food allergy request.

APPROPRIATE USE OF WORDS

There are a few words and statements I want to address in this section that will help you manage your guests' expectations.

- Gluten-free or allergen-free vs. No gluten added or No allergen added
- Need vs. request

What do the words "free of" or "free from" mean? One of the definitions in *Webster's Dictionary* is "not subject to or affected by (a specified thing, typically an undesirable one [substance])." If you plan on referring to any of your menu items as gluten-free or allergen-free you are making a claim that these foods are 100% free of a specific allergen. The Food and Drug Administration (FDA) still has not provided a definition for gluten-free and may never define allergen-free. To claim a product is gluten-free by manufacturing standards, it has to contain less than 20 parts per million (ppm) of gluten. With the possibility of cross-contact during preparation or manufactured products containing an allergen by mistake, can you guarantee this statement is true? If you cannot make this guarantee, do not write the word "free" on your documents or menu. The only time I suggest using the word "free" is to describe a packaged product that is produced by a manufacturer that makes the product in a dedicated allergen-free or gluten-free kitchen, or it carries a certification logo by a recognized authority such as the Gluten-Free Certification Organization (GFCO; www.gfco.org). These products have been tested before they are sold and can carry this guarantee. As long as the package is not opened before serving, it is considered safe and allergen-free. Once you open the package that claim is negated.

Stating "no gluten added" or "no egg added" indicates that the specified allergen was not added to the food. I know it sounds like a play on words but this is the best way to legally communicate product

JJ's Seafood Bar and Grill	
Product Information Sheet	
The following are standard products available at our restaurant. **Always ask to speak to a chef or manager about our products. **Vendors, products, and ingredients may change. **Ingredient labels are available upon request.	
Product	**Allergen Information from Manufacturers Label**
Hot dog bun	Contains milk, soy, wheat
Hamburger bun	Contains milk, soy, wheat
White bread	Contains wheat
Whole wheat bread	Contains soy, wheat
French fries	Pre-fried in soybean oil
Fryer oil	100% soybean oil
Chicken nuggets	Contains egg, milk, soy, wheat
Chicken strips	Contains egg, milk, soy, wheat
Hot dogs	Frozen, contains milk, soy
Hamburgers	Fresh, all-beef
Chicken breast	Fresh, all-natural
Macaroni and cheese	Contains egg, milk, wheat

FIGURE 5.3
PRODUCT INFORMATION SHEET(S).

> If you find a product not on this list, please ask to speak to a chef or manager prior to you visit for product information.
>
> *Disclaimer:* Our company has used reasonable efforts to prevent the introduction of the allergen of concern into the food through close attention during our sourcing, preparation, and handling processes. However, please be advised that you have to use your own individual discretion on making an informed decision based on the information we have provided you. Our company cannot guarantee that allergens may not have been introduced during another stage of the food chain process or even inadvertently by us.

FIGURE 5.3 (CONTINUED)

information to your guests. It is still ultimately up to the guests to make the final decision on ordering any food they choose to eat.

For many years I thought the word *need* was an appropriate word to use when describing special dietary needs. The correct term that should be used is *request*. Why? The definition of *need* means "something that is required because it is essential or very important" verses *request*, which means "an act of asking politely or formally for something".

In this situation, if a guest made their need known to you, you would have to accommodate their need. If they made a request you would have the opportunity to do your best to meet their request. A good example of this is a time when I had a guest request all organic foods for his meal. The guest indicated that he would only eat organic products because of his food allergies.

Our policies did not allow us to purchase organic foods that were not currently on our product list. We could not purchase food from a grocery store, and we did not allow guests to bring their own products for the chef to prepare. We provided the guest with a list of all-natural meats and other foods we did have available. We informed the guest that we would take extra care in preparing and handling the food and that he could bring in his own items that did not require a chef to prepare. With these choices, the guest had a few options. Since the person in the party was only allergic to milk, eggs, peanuts, strawberries, and kiwi, the guest did not really "need" the organic food but was accustomed

To provide you and your family with the best dining experience, please enter your information in the appropriate sections.			
Contact Information			
Contact Person's Name			
Daytime Phone Number			
Evening Phone Number			
E-mail Address			
Date and Time of Visit			
Guest Name with Food Allergy			
Indicate if the guest with the allergy is an adult or child (please provide child(s) age)			
		Adult	Child	Age
	#1			
	#2			
	#3			
	#4			

FIGURE 5.4
DIETARY DATA SHEET.

Type of Allergy or Dietary Request				
	#1	#2	#3	#4
Egg				
Milk/Casein/Dairy				
Peanut				
Tree Nuts				
Fish				
Shellfish				
Soy				
Wheat				
Celiac Disease/Gluten				
Diabetic				
Other				

Other Food Allergies	Foods That Can Be Eaten

Additional Information

Do You Wish a Return Phone Call?	Our company has used reasonable efforts to prevent the introduction of the allergen of concern into the food through close attention during our sourcing, preparation, and handling processes. However, please be advised that you have to use your own individual discretion on making an informed decision based on the information we have provided you. Our company cannot guarantee that allergens may not have been introduced during another stage of the food chain process, or even inadvertently, by us.
Yes No	
Best Time to Reach You	

FIGURE 5.4 (CONTINUED)

To provide you and your family with the best dining experience, please enter your information in the appropriate sections.			
Contact Information			
Contact Person's Name	John Smith		
Daytime Phone Number	123-213-3333		
Evening Phone Number			
E-mail Address	John.smith@foodallergy.ca		
Date and Time of Visit	May 20, 2010		
Guest Name with Food Allergy	Sarah and John		
Indicate if the guest with the allergy is an adult or child (please provide child(s) age)			
		Adult	**Child**	**Age**
	#1	John		
	#2		Sarah	6
	#3			
	#4			

FIGURE 5.5

DIETARY DATA SHEET, COMPLETED.

Type of Allergy or Dietary Request				
	#1	#2	#3	#4
Egg				
Milk/Casein/Dairy				
Peanut				
Tree Nuts				
Fish		×		
Shellfish		×		
Soy				
Wheat				
Celiac Disease/Gluten	×			
Diabetic				
Other		×		

Other Food Allergies	Foods That Can Be Eaten
Sarah is allergic to all berries and mangos.	John is not a picky eater and can eat anything as long as it does not contain any wheat, barley or rye and their by-products. Sarah likes baked chicken, vegetables, and ice cream.

Additional Information
Want to talk to the chef before dining to discuss menu options.

Do You Wish a Return Phone Call?			Our company has used reasonable efforts to prevent the introduction of the allergen of concern into the food through close attention during our sourcing, preparation, and handling processes. However, please be advised that you have to use your own individual discretion on making an informed decision based on the information we have provided you. Our company cannot guarantee that allergens may not have been introduced during another stage of the food chain process, or even inadvertently, by us.
Yes √		No	
Best Time to Reach You			
After 6:00 pm Monday, Wednesday, and Friday			

FIGURE 5.5 (CONTINUED)

FOOD ALLERGY CHECKLIST				
TABLE		SERVER		
DATE		MANAGER OR CHEF ON DUTY		
TIME				
FOOD ALLERGEN				
	MILK		FISH	OTHER
	EGGS		SHELLFISH	
	PEANUT		SOY	
	TREE NUTS		WHEAT	
	GLUTEN		CORN	
MENU ITEMS SERVED TO GUEST				

CHECKLIST REMINDERS	YES	NO
Were all of the allergies recorded on the checklist?		
Were cross-contact issues discussed?		
Was the order confirmed with the chef or manager?		

Keep a copy on file for 30 days in chef's/manager's office.
Internal use only. Do not give a copy to the guest.

Allergy Chefs, Inc. Copyright 2009.

FIGURE 5.6
FOOD ALLERGEN NOTEBOOK. (©2009 ALLERGY CHEFS, INC.)

to eating all organic foods. In the end, we were able to meet the guest's "request" and the guest was satisfied.

COMMUNICATION BY PHONE

Mentioned earlier in this chapter, people sometimes only hear what they want to hear, especially during a phone conversation. It is difficult to convey important information to a guest over the phone and it is equally as hard to collect guest information. That is why I prefer written documents. If you decide to include information by phone, here are a few suggestions.

If you have a phone tree (a system that prompts a caller to push 1 to get to xyz), you can set up a separate phone number or line just to receive food allergy or special dietary requests. This will alert any guest calling about this special service, which can be a plus to your business. Include in the message:

• Specific hours of operation
• Your company Web site or e-mail address
• Request that the guest leave a phone number or e-mail address for follow-up
• When the guest should receive a return phone call

This may seem like a lot of information for a phone message but it can save both the guest and team member valuable time.

If you handle requests at the restaurant without prior correspondence, you can include this information on the phone as well. Here is an example of what to say:

> Most special dietary requests can be accommodated at our dining location. Please make sure to notify the podium or reservation desk attendant of your food allergy or special dietary request prior to being seated. They will notify the person-in-charge of your dietary request and someone will speak with you at your table.

I have found this works well for some guests because there are still people who do not have a computer or do not know how to use one.

So it is important to have a variety of ways to communicate with your guests. This will help reduce their anxiety and let them know that you really get it.

DEVELOP EASY TO UNDERSTAND MESSAGE POINTS

Easy to understand message points should be simple statements that are directed to your team members and guests. These statements will explain what to do, how to do it, and why it should be done. Here are some suggestions for your team members:

- "If a guest tells you someone in their party has a food allergy, notify a leader."
- "Always refer to the food label if there are questions about ingredients."
- "Always take food allergy requests seriously."
- "Do not use common cooking equipment like fryers, grills, and griddles."

Here are some examples that can be directed to your guests:

- "Contact the restaurant at least one week in advance of your dining reservation to talk to a chef about menu options for your allergic guest."
- "Always ask for a chef or manager upon arrival to our restaurants."
- "Ask to read food labels if you have a question about product or menu ingredients."
- "Bring a list of foods you can eat to help the chef decide on the best options for your meal."

There are a few chain restaurants, such as Burger King, Boston Market, and California Pizza Kitchen, that offer easy-to-understand message points and list the allergens on their menu offerings. The benchmark for the industry is Walt Disney World Resorts in Orlando, Florida, and Disneyland in Anaheim, California, where they have established a solid process that makes a food allergic guest's dining experiences magical.

MONITOR FEEDBACK FROM OPERATORS AND GUESTS

As your food allergy program grows, which it will, the special diets manager will need to continue to monitor feedback from the operators and guests. By listening to the feedback, asking questions, and following up with the operators and guests, the special diets manager will be able to make improvements to the program that will benefit everyone.

LIABILITY COST AND THE BOTTOM LINE

There are many costs to running your own food service operation from food and beverage to linens, disposables, chemicals, utilities, labor, liability insurance, and so on. As an operator, you are responsible for your team members' actions while they are at work. Mistakes on the part of one of your team members can be very costly in terms of lawsuits, reputation, and repeat business.

In *Serving the Allergic Guest: Increasing Profit, Loyalty and Safety*, written by Joanne Schlosser of the Food Allergy Awareness Institute, there are examples of not properly handling a food allergic guest request and the cost to the food service establishment and to the guest.

> A 34-year-old man asked a waitress in a Chinese restaurant if the egg rolls were fried in peanut oil, citing his peanut allergy. She assured him that peanut oil was not used. He died 90 minutes later. While no peanut oil was used, the restaurant used peanut butter to seal the ends of the egg roll. This resulted in a $450,000 settlement.
>
> In a similar case, a culinary school was ordered to pay damages of $434,000 to a family of a 27-year-old for negligence in his death. He ordered a vegetarian egg roll but was served one containing shrimp, which caused him to have a fatal allergic reaction.[1]

Real Life Experience: Won't Dine There Again

When my son was a toddler, we went to a popular local chain restaurant for brunch. We brought most of his food along with us but management informed us that they could serve him sliced watermelon. I asked them to have the chef prepare some fresh watermelon. The server assured me that it would not be contaminated with banana or kiwi, two fruits my son is allergic to. Well, after my son had a few bites, his eyes started watering, his mouth got red, and hives started to appear on his face and arms. Luckily, we carried antihistamine with us and gave some to him. The reaction subsided, but our meal was ruined. Cross-contact had happened during the preparation of his fruit. Now we were very nervous, since you never know how a reaction will progress once it starts.

We had to leave without eating our meal. I was so upset about the reaction and that such a small step (cutting up safe fruit with a clean knife and cutting board) could have prevented this. We never, ever go back to this restaurant chain, even if we're dining without my son. I make sure to warn my friends and support group members to be careful if they go eat at this restaurant chain.

Gina Clowes

These are just three examples of what can happen if you do not spend time properly training your staff on food allergy awareness and safety.

COMMUNICATION PROCESS FLOW

Once you have everything in place, the communication process flow (Figure 5.7) should look like this:

1. The guest contacts the dining location and indicates he has a food allergy or special dietary request.
2. The team member handling the call will direct the guest to the Special Diets line to talk to the dietary department.

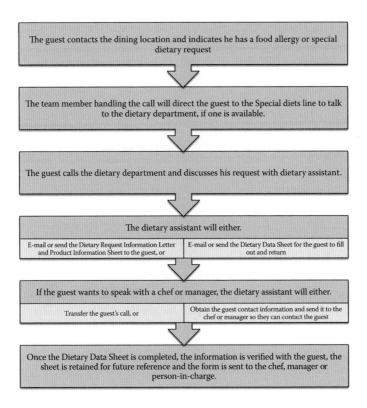

FIGURE 5.7

COMMUNICATION FLOW PROCESS.

3. The guest calls the dietary department and discusses his request with a dietary assistant.
4. The dietary assistant will either:
   a. E-mail or send the Dietary Request Information Letter and Product Information Sheets for the guest to review, or
   b. E-mail or send the Dietary Data Sheet for the guest to fill out and return.
5. If the guest wants to speak with a chef or manager, the dietary assistant will either:
   a. Transfer the guest's call, or
   b. Obtain the guest contact information and send it to the chef or manager so they can contact the guest.

6. Once the Dietary Data Sheet is completed, the information is verified with the guest, the sheet is retained for future reference, and it is sent to the chef, manager, or person in charge. This information will provide them with important information concerning the guest's dietary request.

CHAPTER REVIEW

Before implementing a food allergy program, a special diets committee should be assembled to collect information on current trends in your business. This information will provide the special diets manager in his or her development of communication documents and message points to be shared with the guests and team members. With the proper training and continual monitoring of feedback from both the guest and team members, your food allergy program will continue to improve and provide the safest dining experience for the food allergic guest.

ENDNOTE

1. Joanne Schlosser, MBA, *Serving the Allergic Guest: Increasing Profit, Loyalty and Safety*. (Scottsdale, AZ: Food Allergy Awareness Institute: 2000), 70.

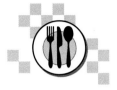

CHAPTER 6

Service Management

A very important aspect about service is having a process or guideline for each step, from greeting guests as they approach the podium to taking their food and beverage order, ringing in the ticket, serving drinks, delivering the food to the table, and checking back with guests throughout their meal. These processes are your established restaurant standards and it is vital that they are written down and properly communicated to every team member.

A process is vital when it comes to handling a food allergy request. There is no room for error. One mistake can lead to unpleasant circumstances. A mistake can cause severe injury or even death to a guest and might possibly lead to litigation.

As was discussed in Chapter 5, "Building a Communication Process," the best communication process can be in place but there can be times when a piece of information is not passed along. This failure of communication may not always be due to the server or chef not communicating correctly but from the guest. Communication is a two-way street and both the guest and food service team have to take responsibility for their part.

THE GUESTS' RESPONSIBILITY

The guests should provide as much information as possible about their food allergy or special diet before their dining experience. Contacting the restaurant to collect information on the level of the staff's food allergy awareness, and willingness to accommodate their request, will help prepare them and the operators for the visit. Upon their arrival to the restaurant, they should notify the podium attendant of their dietary request and ask to speak to a manager or chef before placing their order. They should not assume that the server will be able to answer all of their questions and should make sure that a person in charge is involved with the menu selection.

Real Life Experience: Reputation Isn't Everything

Even at a restaurant chain that has a great reputation for handling food allergies, there is still an obligation on our part to check and double check if something doesn't seem right. My son orders plain hamburgers, and I teach him to look at them. There should not be a trace of cheese (which we've had). Most parents have inadvertently served or almost served their child something unsafe over the years. It's human error.

Gina Clowes

FOOD ALLERGY TRAINING

A few years ago there was little training on food allergies, but now there are several companies and associations that offer food allergy training. The Food Allergy & Anaphylaxis Network (FAAN) is one of the associations that works closely with school, health, food industry, and service professionals to help educate them on food allergy awareness and service.

One of the training tools that FAAN offers is called the 4 R's. I believe these steps can help any food service establishment implement a

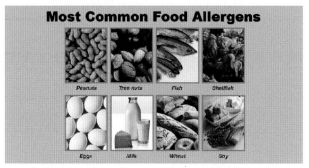

FIGURE 6.1
FOOD ALLERGY POSTER.

successful food allergy-training program. This information can be found on FAAN's restaurant food allergy poster (Figure 6.1). The 4 R's are:

- *Refer* the food allergy concern to the chef, manager, or person in charge.
- *Review* the food allergy with the guest and check ingredient labels.
- *Remember* to check the preparation procedure for potential cross-contact.
- *Respond* to the guest and inform them of your findings.[1]

I have trained hundreds of food service professionals using the 4 R's and have heard of, and personally experienced successful dining experiences when these steps are followed. In the following chapters, I will use the 4 R's to illustrate ways to use them effectively for both front-of-the-house (FOH) and back-of-the-house (BOH) team members.

THE 4 R'S FOR THE FRONT OF THE HOUSE

The front-of-the-house team's success is based on the successful use of the first R: refer the food allergy concern to the chef, manager, or person in charge. It is very important for a person in charge to know that there is a food allergic guest in the establishment. There may be times when a FOH staff member will try to take responsibility, thinking he or she is doing the guest a favor, and handle the request without help. Many FOH staff members do not know enough about kitchen procedures and ingredients to correctly answer basic food allergy questions. There have been many documented experiences that did not turn out well and reflected poorly on the establishment. Due to the increase in food allergies, thorough training and testing on all menu ingredients will ensure that all staff members are prepared to answer guest questions.

STEP 1: REFER THE FOOD ALLERGY CONCERN TO THE CHEF, MANAGER, OR PERSON IN CHARGE

- Podium or the reception desk—When a guest indicates that someone in their party has a food allergy, the podium attendant should:
  - Acknowledge the guest's allergy request.
  - Ask the guest if they contacted the dietary department or restaurant prior to their visit. If so, ask them if they have their information with them.
  - If a seating ticket is used, indicate the allergy on the seating ticket, with any information already known or previously documented. This provides valuable information, such as the table number, date, and time of the guest's dining experience. This ticket should be kept because it contains information that may be needed later if there was an issue. The information on

the ticket will inform the server that there is a guest at the table with a food allergy.
  • Notify management immediately.
• Server—When a guest indicates that someone in their party has a food allergy, the server should:
  • Acknowledge the guest with the allergy. Talk directly with the person providing the information, even if it is a young child or teenager. Many parents are allowing their kids to talk about their allergies to help them take charge of the situation and build confidence.
  • If the guest requests to speak to a manager or chef, notify one before taking an order. This will provide the guest with the assurance that a manager will be notified and will be involved in their dining experience.
• If the guest indicates that you should take the drink order, notify a manager, chef, or the person in charge as soon as the drink order it completed. Food allergic guests do not want to be treated differently and wants everyone in the party to have a good time. Guests want to fit in, not be singled out and yet be reassured that their dining experience is pleasurable and safe.

Stop!: At this point a manager or chef should be meeting with the guest to discuss menu options. I do not recommend the server discussing menu options or taking the food order. A chef or manager should take the order and this information should be written down so nothing is missed.

Real Life Experience: Be Discrete and Show the Guest Respect

At some restaurants, the servers make an embarrassing fuss over the person with food allergies by asking, "Well, what are your food allergies?" My son doesn't want to list or have me list all of his food allergies in front of a crowd.

Gina Clowes

The Food Allergy & Anaphylaxis Network | Chef Card Template

This is an interactive PDF that will allow you to type your allergens directly onto the chef card. To view the fields where you may enter information, click the "Highlight Fields" box in the upper right corner of this window.

WARNING! I am severely allergic to _____

In order for me to avoid a **life-threatening reaction**, I **must avoid** all foods that contain these ingredients:

Please ensure that my food does not contain any of these ingredients, and that any utensils and equipment used to prepare my meals, as well as prep surfaces, are thoroughly cleaned prior to use. **THANK YOU for your cooperation.**

© 2006, The Food Allergy & Anaphylaxis Network, www.foodallergy.org.

How to use your chef card:
In addition to asking a lot of questions about ingredients and preparation methods, many food-allergic teens and adults carry a "chef card" with them that outlines the foods that they must avoid. The card is presented to the chef or manager for review and serves as a reminder of the food allergy.

Print your chef card on brightly colored paper so that it will stand out in a restaurant's hectic atmosphere. Laminate your card to protect it from getting stained. Be sure to make several copies of your chef card so that if you forget to get it back, you have extra copies available.

[PRINT]   [CLEAR]

WARNING! I am severely allergic to _____

In order for me to avoid a **life-threatening reaction**, I **must avoid** all foods that contain these ingredients:

Please ensure that my food does not contain any of these ingredients, and that any utensils and equipment used to prepare my meals, as well as prep surfaces, are thoroughly cleaned prior to use. **THANK YOU for your cooperation.**

© 2006, The Food Allergy & Anaphylaxis Network, www.foodallergy.org.

WARNING! I am severely allergic to _____

In order for me to avoid a **life-threatening reaction**, I **must avoid** all foods that contain these ingredients:

Please ensure that my food does not contain any of these ingredients, and that any utensils and equipment used to prepare my meals, as well as prep surfaces, are thoroughly cleaned prior to use. **THANK YOU for your cooperation.**

© 2006, The Food Allergy & Anaphylaxis Network, www.foodallergy.org.

FIGURE 6.2

FOOD ALLERGY CHEF CARD.

When discussing menu options with the guest it is important to let guests explain all of their food allergies and concerns before taking their order. People with food allergies have a high level of anxiety and want to make sure you understand all of their needs before taking their order. The guests might also give you a food allergy chef card (Figure 6.2), often

ICANEAT™ APP FOR IPHONES, IPOD TOUCH, AND IPAD

Technology is amazing and is affecting every facet of our lives. AllergyFree Passport® partnered with Apple® to create the iCanEat™ application that provides allergen information of certain menu items from a variety of chain restaurants, including Arby's, Boston Market, Burger King, and McDonald's. Your restaurant may be on this list. If you are approached by a guest with the iCanEat™ program in hand, it is best to notify a manager to review the guest's request and double check ingredient statements. A product may have changed or was substituted by the vendor.

called dining cards by food allergic guests (see TriumphDining.com, AllergyFreePassport.com, or FAAN.org), that will provide you with important information that should be given to the chef. A copy of this card is an excellent document to clearly assist the back of the house during the food preparation. It should also be kept on file for repeat visits.

STEP 2: REVIEW THE FOOD ALLERGY WITH THE GUEST AND CHECK INGREDIENT LABELS

- Once a guest informs you of his or her allergies, clarify the guest's food allergies by repeating the allergies back to the guest and writing it down. This is to ensure the guest that you heard him or her correctly. By writing it down you will not forget any details before placing the order or talking to the chef, plus you have a written record of the conversation.
- Document all of the food allergies on a server's ticket or on a Food Allergen Notebook Checklist Sheet. Refer to Chapter 5 for a sample of the checklist.
- Ask the guest what foods he or she usually eats. This is probably one of the most important questions to ask. Knowing what the guest usually eats will make it easier to suggest a menu item that can be prepared for the guest safely. It is not as important to the guest to have a fancy meal as it is to have a safe meal he or she can enjoy.

If servers are taking the order, they should consult with the chef or manager about the menu item that would be appropriate for the guest to eat. *Do not suggest any menu items unless you are 100% sure it does not contain the food allergen mentioned by the guest.* Sometimes menu items contain subingredients that represent certain food allergens that you are not familiar with, such as casein equaling milk or albumin equaling egg. These menu items may also be cooked on shared equipment with other menu items containing food allergens.

Real Life Experience: Never Guess

Never, ever guess when a guest asks about an ingredient. Even if it does not make sense to you, the chef may have a last-minute secret to enhance the flavor of a dish or sauce. Nuts, seafood, dairy, wheat, mustard and more have been known to hide in the most unexpected dishes. When you're asked, ask the chef to find out for sure.

Gina Clowes

STEP 3: REMEMBER TO CHECK THE PREPARATION PROCEDURES FOR POTENTIAL CROSS-CONTACT

- If you are unsure of how a menu item is prepared in the kitchen, check with the chef before making any suggestions. There are many areas in the kitchen where cross-contact can occur, for example, shellfish fried in the same oil as french fries. Menu items that contain certain allergens may be prepared on the same equipment of the menu item that the server suggested.
- If you are unsure of the ingredients in a packaged food, provide guests with the package label for them to review. Remember, food allergic guests are the experts on their food allergy and what foods they are allergic to. They will be able to understand words that are unfamiliar to you on ingredient labels; so let the guests review the label(s) to make sure there are not hidden ingredients in the product.

- Ask the food allergic guest if they have any other dietary concerns. This is a very important step because many guests are so concerned with their food allergies, they forget to tell you about other sensitivities that can make them sick. My experience with this happened when a guest with allergies to milk, eggs, peanuts, tree nuts, and melons left out other food sensitivities. I had written down the allergies and when I was confirming it with the guest I asked again, "Are there any other food allergies or sensitivities I should know about?" The guest said, "Oh, I almost forgot, I am sensitive to onions and garlic." Well, that is a pretty important ingredient in cooking and was almost in every menu item we had. I asked her how sick she would get and she said, "Well, I can be up all night with severe indigestion and heartburn." That was enough for me to inform the guest that I could create something for her without these items too, but the dish would be very simple. She was fine with this and appreciated my thoroughness. That is why it is good idea to double check.

STEP 4: RESPOND TO THE GUESTS AND INFORM THEM OF YOUR FINDINGS

- After reviewing the ingredient statements, checking preparation methods, and confirming the menu options with the chef, manager, or person in charge, respond to the guest and inform them of your findings. If the guest agrees upon the menu options follow these remaining steps.
  - Document the menu options that have been agreed upon in the food allergy notebook (see Figure 6.3).
- Confirm all of the information that is written down with the guest before placing the order. This is the final check to ensure that you and the guest have the same information and the guest is making an informed decision.

STEP 5: DELIVERING THE TICKET TO THE KITCHEN

- Confirm the order with the expeditor or chef before placing the order. This will inform the chef that the order is being placed

FOOD ALLERGY CHECKLIST				
TABLE	45	SERVER	Fred	
DATE	5/19/2010	MANAGER OR CHEF ON DUTY		
TIME	4:00 pm	John		
FOOD ALLERGEN				
√	MILK		FISH	OTHER
√	EGGS		SHELLFISH	Peas
√	PEANUT		SOY	
√	TREE NUTS		WHEAT	
	GLUTEN		CORN	

MENU ITEMS SERVED TO GUEST
Green salad w/ vinegar and oil dressing. Seared and baked chicken breast/salt and pepper. Steamed Broccoli, roasted herb potatoes

CHECKLIST REMINDERS	YES	NO
Were all of the allergies recorded on the checklist?	√	
Were cross-contact issues discussed?	√	
Was the order confirmed with the chef or manager?	√	

Keep a copy on file for 30 days in chef's/manager's office.
Internal use only. Do not give a copy to the guest.
Allergy Chefs, Inc. Copyright 2010

FIGURE 6.3
COMPLETED FOOD ALLERGEN NOTEBOOK CHECKLIST SHEET. (©2010 ALLERGY CHEFS, INC.)

EXPEDITOR'S RESPONSIBILITIES

If you operation has an expeditor, his or her responsibilities are:

- Confirm the order with the server and contact a chef or manager to review the order.
- Once the order is confirmed, attach the food allergy ticket to the ticket that the server rings in.
- Communicate the appropriate information to the chef or cook preparing the meal.
- Once the meal is prepared, place the allergy ticket with the appropriate plate and make sure the person delivering the food takes the correct plate.
- Keep the food allergy ticket until the end of the day and file it in the chef's or manager's office.

so he or she can start preparing or directing the preparation of the meal.
- When placing the order, highlight the food allergy item with one of the following options:
  - "Do not make, see server."
  - "Do not make, see chef."
  - "Food allergy, see chef." I recommend that this option be placed on your point of sale system. This will provide detailed information including the time the meal was rung in and that it is a food allergy request. This will also alert the culinary team that it will need additional information before preparing this meal.
- Once the ticket is rung in, give the food allergy checklist sheet to the chef or expediter so it can be attached to the ticket that was rung into the kitchen.

STEP 6: PREPARING FOOD TO AVOID CROSS-CONTACT

- In the preparation of any food by a server or other front-of-the-house team member, there are precautions that need to be taken to avoid potential cross-contact to the food allergic guest's food.
  - Food grade, vinyl gloves should be used and removed after each use. Additional glove use may be needed if other foods

will be handled. People working in the service area are constantly touching plates, silverware, countertops, and utensils that may expose them to food allergens that can be carried over to the food allergic guest's plate or food. If wearing gloves seems unrealistic, then team members should wash their hands with warm, soapy water for 20 seconds to remove any food allergens before handling any plate, utensil, or food for the guest.

- If a plate of food is prepared incorrectly and is delivered to the guest containing a food allergen, the offending food simply *cannot be removed* from the plate! The plate of food is now contaminated with the food allergen and the entire plate has to be sent to the dish station. A new plate of food has to be prepared from scratch.
  - Examples of this are:
    - Croutons, cheese, nuts added to a salad
    - Whipped cream in a coffee drink
    - Butter or sour cream on a baked potato
- Service area utensils are commonly shared by other servers and may have been used to handle other food items. This will cause the utensil and bulk food item to be contaminated by a food allergen. Do not use ingredients from the common service area such as salad ingredients. The chef or kitchen manager should provide new ingredients.
  - Other examples of utensil cross-contact are:
    - Ladles for soups and dressings
    - Tongs for salad ingredients
    - Portion scoops for ice cream
- Condiment containers (squeeze bottle vs. open tops)

STEP 7: PICKING UP THE FOOD FROM THE KITCHEN

- Confirm the order with the chef and make sure the order matches the food on the plate.
- Avoid the use of a garnish because it may contain a food allergen the guest is allergic to.
- *To avoid cross-contact*, do not stack plates on top or next to the plate for the food allergic guest. Deliver this plate separately to the guest. If you need help, have a manager assist in delivering the plate.

- Confirm the order with the guest to make sure it is prepared correctly.
- Serve all sauces and sides on a separate plate.
- Return to the table in a few minutes to check on the guest.

MANAGER DUTIES

Although it is not always realistic for a chef or manager to personally handle a guest food allergy request, it is still important that the manager be involved.

- If a FOH team member informs you that there is a guest with a food allergy, you should immediately talk to the guest.
- Assist the server with the food allergy request.
- If you are taking the order, follow steps 2 through 5 and 7.
- If you are not taking the order, double check with the kitchen during the preparation of the food.
- Assist the server with delivering the food to the guest.
- Check back with the guests after they have eaten. Guests love this!
- Ask guests for their contact information so you can contact them the regarding their dining experience. This will really let the guests know you are genuinely concerned about their experience and this can help to encourage them to return to your establishment.
- Keep the most frequently asked questions about allergies/preferences in the point of sale or OpenTable system (or file-card system) to track their visits and offer a smoother dining experience upon their return.
- Keeping a copy of the guest's Food Allergy Chefs Card on file is also an excellent idea to ease the guest's subsequent visits.

LOCAL GUESTS ARE GOOD FOR BUSINESS

Guests with food allergies are extremely loyal and do not eat out often. If they find a restaurant that takes their request seriously and they can get a good, safe meal, you will have a loyal customer. Many of them belong to support groups and will tell other group members about their dining experience and recommend your restaurant to them. This may in turn increase your business.

Real Life Experience: Service Gone Bad

We took my son out with our grandparents and some friends to a steakhouse chain restaurant that is supposed to be allergy friendly. I called the chef ahead of time to determine if they could serve us and we planned a safe meal that they said they could make for him.

When we were seated at our table the waitress arrived and said, "Which one of you has the allergies?" I wonder if she would have said, "Which one of you is the diabetic?" It was just very strange and I could see my son shrinking down in his seat. I placed my son's order with her first then the rest of our party ordered.

She brought out the salads but my son's salad was topped with Parmesan croutons and red onion. I explained to her that my son could not have a salad with croutons and she said she'd prepare another one. When she arrived with the next salad and I noticed it had crumbs in it! Someone must have just taken off the croutons. I kept the salad at the table this time. The server finally brought us a new one with just romaine lettuce. By now everyone else had finished their salads.

She finally brought out everyone's entrees except my son's. After a few minutes his steak was delivered. It was almost completely charred. They said the cooks were not used to cooking steaks in a pan, something we had requested because they cook seafood on their grill. My son's steak was so overdone it could hardly be cut. My son did not eat the steak. She also served him a baked potato coated with butter! The potato had to be sent back. I can't even recall if he ever got a "safe" baked potato. It was like there was a neon "food allergy" sign over his head but even with that, they could not get it right.

Gina Clowes

CHAPTER REVIEW

There are many details that front-of-the-house team members need to remember for their daily tasks but none are more important than the 4 R's of food allergy service. They should always *refer* the food allergy request to a leader and assist with the service of the guest. If they take the order, they should *review* the food allergy request with the guest and document information about the order along with reviewing any ingredient statements with the guest. They should always *review* the order with the chef before placing the order. They should *remember* to check for cross-contact of any utensils or food that they serve to the guest. Finally they should *respond* to the guest with any information the guest requested or the information they receive from the chef or manager before placing the order. By following this and the other steps in this chapter, the FOH staff should be properly prepared to serve guests with food allergies with confidence and success.

ENDNOTE

1. The Food Allergy & Anaphylaxis Network, The 4 "R's," 2005, http://www.foodallergy.org (accessed April 25, 2010).

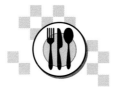

CHAPTER 7

Kitchen Management

Working in today's food service kitchen is very different from what it was years ago. The cost of labor, reduction, and lack of skilled kitchen personnel have forced more chefs to start using premade soups, stocks, and sauces; precut fruits and vegetables; and more convenience foods than ever before. This can make it difficult for chefs or managers to know exactly what ingredients and subingredients are in their menu items because a lot of their dishes are no longer made from scratch. They are relying on vendor product information sheets and labels for ingredient accuracy.

The flow of food is a path that food follows from receiving, storage, preparation, cooking, cooling, reheating, holding, and setup to serving. This flow should be analyzed and reviewed often to make sure it is following safe food-handling guidelines that the Food and Drug Administration (FDA) calls HACCP (hazard analysis and critical control points).

THE FLOW OF FOOD

For more information on the flow of food and food preparation processes visit FDA.gov and search for "Chapter 2—The Process Approach for Managing Food Safety: A Manual for the Voluntary Use of HACCP Principles for Operators of Food Service and Retail Establishments."

Making kitchen management more challenging is the increase of food allergy and special dietary requests. More guests are asking questions like:

- What ingredients are in this menu item?
- How is that menu item prepared?
- Is the chicken free-range and antibiotic-free?
- Where does the seafood originate?
- Is the produce organic?
- Is this dish vegetarian or vegan?

Some of these questions may be easily answered but during busy meal periods, questions like this may take some time to answer and the information may be hard to find. Rushing to find the answers may cause incorrect or incomplete information being shared with a guest, which could cause the guest to get sick. You have probably heard some of these questions before. That is why it is important to develop standard operating procedures (SOPs) to equip your operation to be able to answer these questions.

This chapter is designed to help chefs, managers, or the person in charge of kitchen operations develop an SOP based on HACCP principles and the 4 R's (refer, review, remember, respond) that were discussed in Chapter 6. First, HACCP will be reviewed and a plan will be designed and applied for food allergen control in the kitchen. Then the 4 R's will be applied to the actual preparation and service of a meal once the order is taken and sent to the kitchen.

HACCP PLAN FOR FOOD ALLERGEN SAFETY

As defined by the FDA,

> HACCP or Hazard Analysis and Critical Control Points is a management system that addresses food safety through the analysis and control of biological, chemical, and physical hazards from raw material production, procurement and handling, to manufacturing, distribution and consumption of a finished product.[1]

The original concept of HACCP was developed in the early 1960s by the Pillsbury Company while working with NASA and U.S. Army Laboratories[2] and has been applied to many aspects of the food industry. It is fitting that this system be utilized to manage food allergens in the food service kitchen.

Since HACCP was designed to minimize food safety risks in the food processing industry, it is not zero risk and does not eliminate the possibility of a hazard getting into the food product. It is the same with a food allergen. There is not a 100% guarantee that a food allergen will not get into the food that is being prepared. By utilizing the following steps, the possibility can be minimized.

- Step 1: Develop prerequisite programs
- Step 2: Group menu items by allergens
- Step 3: Conduct a hazard analysis
- Step 4: Implement control measures for critical control points
- Step 5: Establish monitoring procedures
- Step 6: Develop corrective actions

STEP 1: DEVELOP PREREQUISITE PROGRAMS

New programs or changes to kitchen procedures must start with a good foundation that will ensure that the program will be sustainable and easily managed. To accomplish this, I suggest implementing the following prerequisite programs prior to fully handling food allergy requests.

- Food allergy training program—Training team members on food allergy awareness, proper communication between the guest and the kitchen, prevention of cross-contact, and appropriate emergency procedures are key elements to the overall program's success.

ADDITIONAL TRAINING RESOURCES

Besides the information presented in this book, resources for training material can be purchased from the Food Allergy & Anaphylaxis Network, the National Restaurant Association, or Allergy Chefs, Inc. More information about these training programs can be found in the Appendix of this book.

- Vendor partnership program—Partner with your vendors to explain your expectations concerning food allergens. Have them supply you with current ingredient statements that contain a full list of ingredients, allergens, and production procedures. Incorporate an SOP concerning notification of product substitution and ingredient changes so that these changes can be properly communicated to your team and guests. If a vendor ceases to produce an item or can no longer guarantee the allergen-free status of ingredients, you have three options:

  1. Seek out another company that can supply you the product
  2. Change the recipe to remove the ingredient
  3. Update the recipe with the current information

- Recipe/process instructions—First, develop a standard recipe format that includes allergen identification. When creating new menu items, identify food allergens and decide if they are needed in the recipe. If the ingredient is not needed or a substitute that is not a major food allergen can be used, you will have a menu item that is a better option for more guests. Second, review cooking procedures to identify the potential of cross-contact from the use of common cooking equipment.

ICIX: MANAGING RISK, COMPLIANCE, AND STANDARDS

A company specializing in ingredient documentation is iCiX. Thousands of customers, including most of the major brands, use the iCiX network to effectively and efficiently manage validated compliance documentation and communication. With iCiX, all members can manage risk and protect their brand at every stage of the supply chain. With iCiX you can be sure that each one of your trading partners lives up to the standards of quality and safety set by your company. iCiX network contains product information that can be tailored to your company needs, especially food allergen information. You can learn more by visiting the Web site www.icix.com.

CROSS-CONTAMINATION VS. CROSS-CONTACT

Cross-contamination is a common factor in the cause of foodborne illness. Microorganisms such as bacteria and viruses from different sources can contaminate foods during preparation and storage. Proper cooking of the contaminated food in most cases will reduce or eliminate the chances of a foodborne illness.

Cross-contact occurs when an allergen is inadvertently transferred from a food containing an allergen to a food that does not contain the allergen. Cooking does not reduce or eliminate the chances of a person with a food allergy having a reaction to the food eaten. This is the main difference between the two statements.

- A good example of this is the use of a flattop grill. During breakfast the grill maybe used to scramble eggs or cook French toast, so the grill would contain egg, milk, and wheat proteins. During lunch, the grill maybe used to toast breads or cook meats. These items may not contain milk or egg proteins but if the grill was not properly cleaned before lunch, the allergens will still be present. These foods would now come in contact with these proteins and be contaminated. This is an example of cross-contact.
- Ingredient/recipe book—There are differences between an ingredient book and a recipe book. An *ingredient book* could contain actual ingredient labels, photocopies of ingredient labels, vendor ingredient statements, or retyped ingredient statements. This type of book can be beneficial when sharing information with the guest but has two major flaws.

1. The inability to update ingredient information in a timely manner.
2. Retyped ingredient statements can be improperly translated.

If someone is dedicated to monitoring product changes or the operation has a static menu with minimal menu changes or product substitutions, an ingredient book may be a good option.

Chef Joel's Breakfast Special

Yield: Four 6 ounce servings
Prep time: 20 minutes
Cook time: 5–7 minutes

This is a recreation of a recipe I learned while working in an Italian restaurant in Fresno, California. It was our best seller and a great dish for anytime of the day. It is usually finished off with parmesan cheese and eggs but it is also good without them.

Allergen	Ingredients	Quantity
	Canola oil	1 ounce
	Fresh garlic, peeled and minced	1 tablespoon
	Yellow or sweet onion, diced	4 ounces
	Ground beef, pork, or chicken	1 pound
	Button or crimini mushrooms, cleaned and sliced	3 ounces
	Frozen chopped spinach, thawed and drained	8 ounces
Eggs	Eggs (optional)	2 each
Milk	Parmesan cheese, grated (optional)	1 ounce

FIGURE 7.1
SAMPLE RECIPE FORMAT 1.

A *recipe book* is common in most, if not all kitchens. Incorporating a standard recipe format to include allergens and vendor ingredient statements will be easier to manage and keep updated. Designate a chef to keep recipes current and have the chef partner with the food handler or receiver and vendors to keep ingredient information current. See Figure 7.1 and Figure 7.2 for two types of recipe formats.

Step	Procedure
1	Heat the oil in a large sauté pan over high heat.
2	Add the garlic and onions; cook, stirring often for 1 minute.
3	Add the ground meat; cook, stirring often until the meat is thoroughly cooked. Do not drain the fat.
4	Add the mushrooms; cook until soft.
5	Loosen up the spinach and mix it into the other ingredients. At this point, the dish can be seasoned with salt and served. If you want to add the eggs and cheese, follow steps 6 and 7.
6	Make a hole in the center of the mixture and add 1 tablespoon of oil.
7	Add the eggs; scramble until completely cooked. Sprinkle with the cheese and mix the ingredients together. Serve immediately.

FIGURE 7.1 (CONTINUED)

Chicken and Tortilla Casserole with Cabot Cheddar Cheese
Allergens: Milk & Soy
Yield: 15 servings

Ingredients

Salsa Verde

1 can (13 oz) tomatillos, drained **(ingredient label upon request)**

1 large yellow onion, peeled and cut into chunks

1 each garlic clove

1 can (4 oz) diced green chilies **(ingredient label upon request)**

1 bunch fresh cilantro, stems removed

2 tablespoons sugar (optional)

Salt and black pepper to taste

Casserole

4 cups shredded cooked chicken, skin removed

1 cup sour cream or tofutti (soy) sour cream **(ingredient label upon request)**

12 each corn tortilla (6-inch diameter), cut into ¼-inch-wide strips **(ingredient label upon request)**

4 cups (1 pound) shredded Cabot Cheddar cheese

1 large ripe avocado, pitted, peeled, and thinly sliced (prepared just before serving)

FIGURE 7.2

SAMPLE RECIPE FORMAT 2.

Method of Preparation

1. Prepare Salsa Verde.
2. In a blender or food processor, combine the tomatillos, onions, garlic, green chilies, and cilantro. Blend until smooth. Adjust with salt, pepper, and sugar if needed.
3. Combine the sour cream to that salsa and blend until smooth.
4. To assemble the casserole, place half of the chicken in a 9-by-13-inch baking dish.
5. Top with half of the salsa/sour cream mixture and spread evenly.
6. Top with half of the tortilla strips and half of the Cabot Cheddar cheese.
7. Repeat layers, using remaining chicken, salsa/sour cream, tortilla strips, and cheese.
8. Cover with foil and bake in a 350°F oven for 40 minutes.
9. Uncover and continue baking until the cheese is bubbly (5 to 10 more minutes).

Presentation or Assembly

1. Remove from the oven and let stand for 10 minutes; then arrange avocado slices on top of casserole.
2. Cut into squares to serve.
3. Top with your favorite salsa and freshly chopped cilantro to create an exciting plated entrée.

Preparation time: about 30 minutes
Baking time: 45 to 50 minutes

FIGURE 7.2 (CONTINUED)

Real Life Experience: Reading Food Labels for Hidden Ingredients

We love labels and don't mind reviewing a recipe. Many times, I've had chefs hand me a label because they weren't sure of the ingredients. I've also read over recipes that they thought were safe but really weren't because the ingredients contained words like "spices" or "natural flavors." Potent allergens like sesame or mustard can hide behind these labels, and we don't take chances like that. Normally, if I want my son to try a product that included "natural flavors" or "spices" on the label, I'd call the manufacturer. When we're out to dinner, I would not take a chance on giving my son a product that contained these ingredients. So while a chef might not give the word "spices" a second thought, I certainly would.

Gina Clowes

STEP 2: GROUP MENU ITEMS BY ALLERGENS

HACCP has a specific way of grouping menu items using the flow of food and three process-specific lists for food preparation.

Process #1: Food preparation with no cook step
Process #2: Food preparation with same day service
Process #3: Complex food preparation[3]

Since cooking does not eliminate food allergens (proteins), these steps do not apply, but the following steps will be helpful in identifying food allergens in menu items and cooking procedures.

- Analyze current recipes to identify known allergens—Once a decision has been made on a recipe format, start reviewing each recipe to identify the top eight food allergens in each recipe. Indicate the allergens on the recipe and categorize the recipes by allergens or by stations, then place them in a recipe book, filing cabinet, or computer file. By categorizing them by station it may help you identify other allergens that are in each station during service. This could pinpoint areas of possible cross-contact and help provide valuable information that can be shared with guests to help them make an informed decision on whether to order that menu item.
- Review ingredient statements of prepared foods from vendors—If prepared foods are used that require you to repackage or heat prior to service, review vendor ingredient statements for hidden allergens. Some products, such as freshly baked bread from a local vendor, may not have an ingredient statement. Request one immediately. By law, all prepared foods must comply with the Food Allergen Labeling and Consumer Protection Act.
- Identify the cooking procedure for each recipe—List the cooking procedure on the recipe and identify what equipment is used in its preparation. If the menu item has multiple cooking steps before it reaches its final presentation, there is the possibility of cross-contact in the preparation steps. See Figure 7.3 for example.

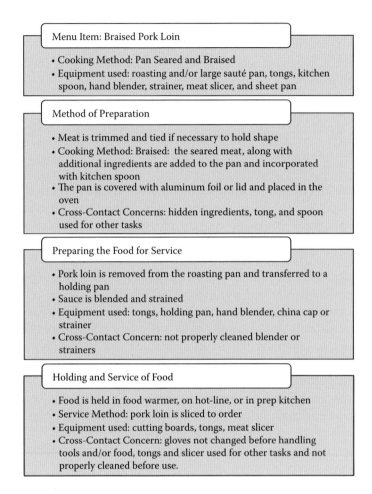

Menu Item: Braised Pork Loin

- Cooking Method: Pan Seared and Braised
- Equipment used: roasting and/or large sauté pan, tongs, kitchen spoon, hand blender, strainer, meat slicer, and sheet pan

Method of Preparation

- Meat is trimmed and tied if necessary to hold shape
- Cooking Method: Braised: the seared meat, along with additional ingredients are added to the pan and incorporated with kitchen spoon
- The pan is covered with aluminum foil or lid and placed in the oven
- Cross-Contact Concerns: hidden ingredients, tong, and spoon used for other tasks

Preparing the Food for Service

- Pork loin is removed from the roasting pan and transferred to a holding pan
- Sauce is blended and strained
- Equipment used: tongs, holding pan, hand blender, china cap or strainer
- Cross-Contact Concern: not properly cleaned blender or strainers

Holding and Service of Food

- Food is held in food warmer, on hot-line, or in prep kitchen
- Service Method: pork loin is sliced to order
- Equipment used: cutting boards, tongs, meat slicer
- Cross-Contact Concern: gloves not changed before handling tools and/or food, tongs and slicer used for other tasks and not properly cleaned before use.

FIGURE 7.3
ANALYSIS OF COOKING PROCEDURES TO IDENTIFY CROSS-CONTACT

STEP 3: CONDUCT A HAZARD ANALYSIS

A hazard analysis is designed to identify the food safety hazards (biological, chemical, and physical) that exist in the flow of food in a food service operation from receiving to service or sale. By identifying the food safety hazard present in your system, you should be able to identify possible control measures that may be implemented to prevent a foodborne illness. Control measures are any actions or activities that can be used to prevent, eliminate, or reduce an identified hazard.[4] In this case, the food safety hazard is a food allergen coming in contact with a menu item before it is served to a guest with a food allergy. Developing a list of questions can help you identify potential hazards in your operation.

- Do we have the proper ingredient statement for each menu item?
- Where can cross-contact occur in the food handling and preparation of each menu item?
- Are utensils, cutting boards, pots, and pans properly cleaned and sanitized?
- Are gloves changed and hands washed before handling food for a guest with food allergies?
- Was the food cooked on common cooking equipment?
- Were the utensils used to handle the food used for something else?

These are a sample of questions for you to use as a starting point. Food service operations run differently so additional questions may arise.

STEP 4: IMPLEMENT CONTROL MEASURES
FOR CRITICAL CONTROL POINTS

The FDA defines a critical control point (CCP) as

> an operational step at which control can be applied and is essential to prevent or eliminate a hazard or reduce it to an acceptable level. If an operational step is the last step at which control can be applied to prevent or eliminate a hazard or reduce it to an acceptable level, then you should consider controlling it as a CCP. If a step later in the process will control the hazards of concern, that step, rather than the one in question, will most likely be a CCP.[5]

The major difference between controlling the introduction of an HACCP-defined food safety hazard and a food allergen is that there is *no acceptable level* of a food allergen that can be present in the food to make it safe.

COMMON OPERATIONAL STEPS

The following information is provided to assist in your decision making as you develop the procedural steps presented in this chapter. Common operational steps focused on eliminating the introduction of food allergens include, but are not limited to, receiving, storing, preparing, cooking, hot and cold holding, assembly/setup/packing, and serving. If your operation is currently following HACCP guidelines, then you are already in a good position to prevent food allergen cross-contact.[6]

Receiving and Storage

Receiving and storage is an important operational step to prevent cross contamination of foods by keeping food out of the temperature danger zone (41°F–135°F) for a specific time (4 hours). It is also important to properly store foods that have common food allergens, such as dairy, egg, and wheat-based products. Keeping these items in a designated area, clearly labeled, can help prevent cross-contact of other foods. Other steps that should be taken are:

- Receivers or food handlers should inform a chef, manager, or person in charge if a vendor substitutes a product so that ingredient/recipe books can be updated with the changes.
- All products should be stored properly and any special dietary products should be handled with care and placed in their appropriate location.
- Review how products are stored or held in the cooking and service area.

Food Preparation

Of all the operational steps, food preparation is where cross-contact can occur most frequently. Since there are many tasks being performed in the kitchen, there is always the possibility of a worker using a cutting board or kitchen tool that has been used for another task and not properly cleaned between use, or not following a cooking procedure correctly, or adding additional ingredients to a recipe. These are some of the details that the chef, manager, or person in charge, has to keep in mind when handling a food allergy request. Here are some other points to consider and review in your operation.

- Review where products are being prepared in the kitchen—Items prepared in a bakery or pastry shop may come in contact with wheat proteins because of the wheat particles floating in the air.
- Review who is preparing the food and what steps are taken to prepare the food—With the downsizing of kitchen staff and high turnover, many cooks are preparing multiple items that may contain a variety of allergens. If they are not following proper preparation procedures or HACCP guidelines, cross-contact of a menu item may occur.
- Ask the cooks how the recipes are prepared—For example, baked chicken wings, tossed with canola oil and seasoned with spices, salt, and pepper, then placed on a sheet pan lined with parchment and baked. A cook may use a spray on the sheet pan in addition to or instead of the parchment paper to keep the food from sticking. There may be an allergenic ingredient in the spray that you are not aware of and could cause someone to have a reaction.
- Latex vs. vinyl gloves—Latex allergies are real. Nonlatex gloves should be used in the food preparation areas. The American Latex Association states that if latex gloves are used to handle food, the food must be washed thoroughly or cooked before serving. This will remove the latex allergen residue.
- Refrigerator doors and handles—Doors and handles are breeding grounds for bacteria and allergens since many employees handle them throughout the day. You should always wash your hands or change gloves after coming in contact with any door handle before touching any food for a guest with food allergies.
- Kitchen tools—You should have designated cutting boards, knives, and utensils for preparing special meals. A specially designed cutting board made by San Jamar called "The Purple Board™" is available with step-by-step instructions and tips. San Jamar also offers an Allergen Saf-T-Zone™ System that includes the board, 10-inch chef's knife, tongs, and stainless steel tongs and turner with the same-colored handles.
- Meat slicer—Be aware of foods prepared on a meat slicer. If the equipment is not properly cleaned between uses, residue from cheese or meats containing additives can be transferred onto other foods prepared on this machine.

LATEX ALLERGY

According to the American Latex Allergy Association, nearly 3 million Americans are allergic to latex.[*] Food service workers are in danger of developing a latex allergy.[7] People with a latex allergy can have cross-reactive allergic reaction with certain fruits and vegetables, which is often referred to as latex-fruit syndrome. I have worked with some food service professionals with a latex allergy including my wife, Mary. The following foods have been identified to cause an allergic reaction in people with a latex allergy. They are listed by the degrees of association to latex or prevalence of allergic reactions.

- High: avocado, banana, chestnut, and kiwi
- Moderate: apple, carrot, celery, melons, papaya, potato, tomato
- Low/undetermined: apricot, cherry, citrus fruits, fig, grape, lychee, mango, nectarine, passion fruit, peach, pear, persimmon, pineapple, strawberry, buckwheat, rye, wheat, coconut, hazelnut, walnut, castor bean, chickpea, soybean, dill, oregano, sage, peppers (cayenne, sweet/bell), shellfish, sunflower seed.[8]

Cooking

As discussed earlier, cooking is an effective operational step to reduce or eliminate biological contamination, but cooking does not eliminate food allergens. Food allergens are proteins that will bind up and lose moisture when cooked but will not be eliminated.

- Create a "food allergen safety zone" to prepare foods that do not contain the top eight food allergens (Figure 7.4). If your kitchen has enough space, set up a station where food can be prepared for special dietary requests. Educate your staff on the importance of this section and have only the chef or the person designated to

---

[*] Because of frequent use of latex.

Kitchen Tools:
San Jamar's Allergen Saf-T-Zone™ tools: 10" chef's knife,
stainless steel tongs and turner all in matching purple to
coordinate with The Purple Board™, along with designated serving plates

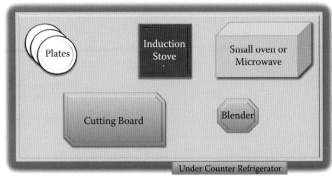

Kitchen Equipment: Induction stove, blender, sauté pans, sauce pan, grill or griddle pan, small oven or microwave

Food:
Unseasoned chicken breast, steaks, or pork, carrots, broccoli, potatoes, pancake mix, gluten-free bread or rolls, Olive oil or herb oil, and vinegar

Beverage & Desserts:
Soy or rice milk, apple juice, individually wrapped cookies or brownies, unsweetened applesauce, soy, coconut or rice milk frozen desserts, and fresh fruit

FIGURE 7.4
FOOD ALLERGEN SAFETY ZONE.

prepare these foods work in this section during service. If team members violate this procedure, you should have disciplinary actions to hold them accountable, just like you would for someone violating a food safety procedure.

• Common cooking equipment should not be used to cook food for an allergic guest unless the equipment is designated to cook only one item or you know exactly what ingredients are prepared using this equipment.

  • Equipment to avoid:
    – Grills
    – Flattop griddles
    – Fryers
    – Tilt skillet
    – Meat slicer
    – Cast iron skillets (unless designated)
    – Waffle irons

- Equipment to use:
  - Individual sauté pans and skillets
  - Individual baking pans with covers or that can be covered with foil
  - Individual grills or griddles to use to prepare pancakes or grilled meats
  - Waffle iron designated to use with a special dietary waffle mix (All-Clad MetalCrafters, LLC)
  - Individual fryer that will only be used for specific items such as french fries or allergen-free chicken nuggets (Fry Daddy™)
  - Individual steamer for steaming vegetables (Oster™ or Black & Decker™)
  - Designate an oven during service for baked items or heating up bread
    - Any item heated in the oven during service should be covered to prevent any foreign particles from touching the food.
    - I use a KitchenAid® countertop oven that works great for cooking small batches of foods. If the food is pre-cooked, it will take less time to prepare.
  - Microwave oven
- Cooking food to order in individual pans and using designated utensils is the safest way to prepare food for a guest with an allergy. This controls what ingredients are added, how the food is prepared, and how it will be served.
- It will take additional time to cook a guest's meal by following these preparation procedures, so it is important to inform the guest that it may take longer to prepare his or her meal.

Holding Food for Service

Now that the food is prepared for service, time should be taken to properly set up each station to prevent cross-contact of prepared foods (Figure 7.5). When food is held for service there is an increased risk for cross-contact caused by personnel, equipment, procedures, or other factors.[9] Review the placement of each item to identify foods containing allergens and arrange them so that when serving or dishing up these

Roasted Herb Potatoes (Allergens–NA)	Cornbread Stuffing (Allergens–wheat & milk)	Citrus Crusted Fish (Allergens–fish, milk, tree nuts, wheat)	Sautéed Vegetables (Allergens–NA)	Seafood Chowder (Allergens–fish, shellfish, milk, wheat)
	Sliced Turkey (Allergens–NA)		Macaroni & Cheese (Allergens–milk, wheat, soy)	Turkey Pan Gravy (Allergens–NA)

Allergen-Free Items			Items with Common Allergens	
Roasted Herb Potatoes (Allergens–NA)	Sliced Turkey (Allergens–NA)	Citrus Crusted Fish (Allergens–fish, milk, tree nuts, wheat)	Extra pan for additional menu item	Cornbread Stuffing (Allergens–wheat & milk)
Sautéed Vegetables (Allergens–NA)	Turkey Pan Gravy (Allergens–NA)		Seafood Chowder (Allergens–fish, shellfish, milk, wheat)	Macaroni & Cheese (Allergens–milk, wheat, soy)

Reduce the amount of potatoes and split this space so it can hold two items. Now this section has foods that do not contain the top 8 food allergens. This can be a convenient way to make a complete meal by offering these items.

FIGURE 7.5

STATION REDESIGN TO REDUCE FOOD ALLERGEN CROSS-CONTACT.

items, particles from the food do not drip or come in contact with other foods. This procedure will also help the cooks use the correct serving utensil for the designated dish.

Set Up, Assembly, and Packing

Set up, assembly, and packing are operational steps used by some retail food establishments that may involve wrapping food items, assembling items onto trays, and packing them for transportation or for display cases. An example of this would be a catering kitchen preparing food that is wrapped, assembled, and placed in portable food carts that is taken to a final holding area for service. Room-service kitchens set up guest trays and place them into portable hot boxes and transport the food to the guest rooms. Food may also be repackaged and labeled to be sold in retail coolers or placed in bulk containers for transportation to another site to be assembled and served.[10]

Along with addressing the potential for bacterial contamination and growth, bare-hand contact with ready-to-eat foods, and proper hand washing, you should consider the following:

- Have a list of ingredients for each menu item available to review, if necessary.
- Keep specially made foods in separate containers and label correctly.
  - For example, if you are serving gluten-free breads or have a plate prepared without milk, nuts, or wheat, these items would be stored separately and correctly labeled.
- Any prepackaged food should have the correct ingredients listed on the label, including the subingredients of combined products such as sauces or spices.

Serving

Serving the food is the final step before the food reaches the guest. All employees should be properly trained to prevent cross-contact at this critical stage. The following steps should be taken:

- Proper hand washing
- Appropriate use of gloves and dispensing utensils
- Control of bare-hand contact with foods
- Designate a special plate or serving tray that is easily identifiable (Corelle® Contours, Edgy, http://www.corelle.com/index.asp?pageId=72)

You could have followed every procedure correctly and prepared the food to meet the guest's dietary concern but it could all be for naught if the wrong food is delivered to the guest and they become sick.

STEP 5: ESTABLISH MONITORING PROCEDURES FOR KITCHEN PREPARATION

Monitoring is observing, checking, or keeping record of a specific operational step in the food process to determine if the critical limits you have established are met. To prevent food allergen cross-contact it is recommended that the critical control points be under control. Monitoring will identify when there is a loss of control or a trend toward a loss of control so corrective action can be taken.[11]

You should establish answers to the following questions:

- What will you monitor?
- How will you monitor?
- When and how often will you monitor?
- Who will be responsible for monitoring?

You will have to establish what you are going to monitor based on the greatest possibility of cross-contact. Using special dietary products or effectively utilizing designated cooking equipment and procedures are very important, and you should determine how you will effectively monitor the proper use for them and when they should be used.

Utilizing tools or other types of equipment or procedures to monitor cross-contact should be utilized. If you currently use a HACCP checklist, it should include additional questions that pertain to food allergen safety. This should be shared with team members so they are aware of the expectation of each step.

Daily monitoring of these procedures can be included as a discussion in your preshift meetings and in your daily inspection of the kitchen. This could become one of your regular routines, but do not become complacent. Food allergies are real and need to be taken seriously.

Monitoring these processes more closely will make you more aware of your kitchen operations, how the food is prepared, and what ingredients are in each menu item. This will enable you to reduce the risk of cross-contact.

STEP 6: DEVELOP CORRECTIVE ACTIONS

Corrective actions are very simple when it comes to food allergens.

- If a menu item ingredient has changed, the information has to be communicated immediately to all team members.
- If a menu item becomes contaminated with a possible allergen, this should be communicated to the wait staff and the product must not be served to a guest

- If a food allergic guest's food item is contaminated with a food allergen or the menu item is incorrectly prepared, the items should be discarded and a fresh one prepared.

Now that we have established the procedural steps to ensure that food allergens can be easily identified in the kitchen, we will review the service steps necessary to execute a food allergy request.

THE 4 R'S FOR THE KITCHEN

The back-of-the-house (BOH) team has the most important part in the whole food allergy process and is responsible for the final preparation of the meal. This is where the majority of the responsibility lies. Let us review the 4 R's before we discuss how they can be applied to the kitchen.

- *Refer* the food allergy concern to the chef, manager, or person in charge.
- *Review* the food allergy with the guest and check ingredient labels.
- *Remember* to check the preparation procedure for potential cross contact.
- *Respond* to the guest and inform them of your findings.

STEP 1: REFER THE FOOD ALLERGY CONCERN TO THE CHEF, MANAGER, OR PERSON IN CHARGE

As a leader, refer does not usually apply to you unless you are a manager and will be referring the food allergy request to a chef. This step may take place at different times. Some guests may contact you before their visit, whereas others will just show up in your dining room during your peak service time. It is hoped you will know beforehand and will be prepared for their visit, so we will start here.

COMMUNICATING WITH GUESTS BEFORE THEIR VISIT

From my experience, most chefs do not come out of the kitchen to talk with a guest unless we are requested. That is left up to the manager.

Times have changed with the awareness of food allergies and special diets, and it is becoming more of a requirement of today's chefs. So it is beneficial if a chef, manager, or person in charge is notified by guests prior to their dining experience.

Guests who contact the restaurant prior to their reservation want to get more details about their options and how food is prepared. What I have learned is guests with food allergies are loyal to brand products, special treatment, and have specific requests concerning food preparation that will keep them safe.

As was described in Chapter 5, "Getting Started," placing a special message on the chef's or manager's voicemail indicating that special dietary requests can be handled has benefits. When guests are directed to call a chef or manager with questions, this message provides them with some reassurance that they contacted the right person and they should be receiving a return call as soon as possible.

When having a conversation with a guest about his or her request, here are some helpful tips.

- Contact the guest when you have time to talk.
  - The call may take some time because the guest will be asking many questions.
- Do not sound rushed.
  - The guest may get the feeling that you are too busy to really listen.
- Have something to document the conversation.
  - Utilize the dietary data sheet found in Chapter 5. The guest may have sent one to the restaurant so use it to add any additional information about their request.
    - You may be asked about the iPhone™, iCanEat™ application for your restaurant. If you are not, have enough information on your company's involvement in this, write down the guest's request, and call them back when you have the correct information.
- Ask my favorite question, "What do you or your child usually eat?"
  - This will help you identify current menu items that could be used or modified.

- If the guest requests a special dietary product, see if a vendor can acquire it for you or find out if your company policy allows you to purchase it from the grocery store.
- If you do not have an answer to one a guest's questions, be honest. If you do not know, you do not know. It is better not to know something then pretend to know the answer and be wrong.
- Show understanding and empathy.

Once the conversation is completed, file the information in a location that can be easily retrieved. Here are three best practices that can help keep this information organized.

- Binder with month and day tabs—Keep any written documents such as the food allergy/dietary request in this binder.
- Daily clipboards—Place information in the kitchen so it can be referred to daily.
- Outlook calendar—If you work with different leaders, add any special requests on everyone's calendar so the person in charge for that meal period will be aware of this guest's request.

PREPARING THE KITCHEN FOR FOOD ALLERGY REQUESTS

As a chef, it is very important to me to have everything in place before starting service. With food allergy requests becoming more prevalent in today's kitchens, it is essential that this procedure be included in daily preparation. As discussed in the Food Allergen HACCP section, there are certain tools and products that should be used to ensure food is prepared safely. Here is a list of items that should be in place before service begins.

1. Documents with daily food allergy requests.
2. Food allergy notebook to write down guest information.
3. Colored-coded utensils and cutting boards to use in the preparation of these meals.
4. Individual sauté or sauce pans.
5. Designated plate to serve prepared foods.
6. Nonlatex gloves.
7. Small cooler or refrigerator to store special products.
8. Designated "food allergen safety zone."

9. Unseasoned meats, vegetables, and starches.
10. Plain olive or canola oil.

STEP 2: REVIEW THE FOOD ALLERGY WITH THE GUEST AND CHECK INGREDIENT LABELS

Now it is service time and you are either in the kitchen or on the floor managing your team and you are notified of a food allergy request, what do you do? You rely on the last three R's to take you through the process. We will discuss two scenarios in reference to step 2. Scenario 1 is when the chef, manager, or person in charge speaks with the guest, and scenario 2 is when the server takes the order and notifies the kitchen.

SCENARIO 1: VISITING THE GUEST AT THE TABLE

1. Once the guest informs you of their allergies, clarify the guest food allergies by repeating them back to the guest. Then ask the guest again if there are any additional food allergies or sensitivities. I have found that some guests are only focused on the major foods they are allergic to and forget to mention other food sensitivities. It is best to know every food allergy or sensitivity so that you can determine the best menu option for him or her.

Real Life Experience: More Food Allergies?

There are allergies to all kinds of different foods: mustard, sesame, lentil, garlic, and banana. We know it sounds strange, but it's true. It's much better for us as the guest to report these allergies to you up front than for an allergic reaction to happen in your restaurant.

Gina Clowes

---

2. Document all food allergies on a standard notebook such as the food allergen notebook found in Chapter 6. This is to ensure that you heard the guest correctly and will not forget any detail about their order.

3. Ask the guest what foods they usually eat. This is one of the most important questions to ask. Knowing what they usually eat will make it easier to suggest a menu item that can be prepared for them safely. You should understand that it is not as important to the guest to have a fancy meal, as it is to have a safe meal they can enjoy with their family.

Real Life Experience: No Pheasant under Glass Please

We don't require pheasant under glass to be happy. We just need a safe meal. If you are just starting in accommodating special dietary needs, come up with a few basic options. Think plain meats, pastas, steamed vegetables or rice. With multiple food allergies, it's better to focus on what they can have. When in doubt, serve sauces and condiments on the side.

Gina Clowes

---

4. Discuss any cooking and handling procedures with the guest concerning their meal.
5. If there are any questions or concerns about ingredients, provide the guest with the package label or an ingredient/recipe book if one is available.
6. Document the menu options you and the guest agreed upon in the notebook.
7. Inform the guest that it may take additional time to prepare their meal since it will probably be made from scratch.
8. Provide the server with the following information:
   a. What the guest is eating.
   b. What they can prepare for the guest.
   c. The needed information so they can ring in the order.

SCENARIO 2: THE SERVER TAKES THE ORDER

1. Review the food allergy with the server.
2. If necessary, review any ingredient labels before suggesting a menu option.
3. Remember to check the preparation procedures for potential cross-contact.

4. Review the menu options with the server.
5. Document the guest's food allergies and menu options on the checklist.
6. Have the server review the food allergies and menu options with the guest before preparing the meal.
7. Once the meal has been confirmed with the guest, have the server ring in the order.

STEP 3: REMEMBER TO CHECK THE PREPARATION PROCEDURE FOR POTENTIAL CROSS-CONTACT

1. Once the meal ticket is ordered, attach the food allergy checklist sheet to the server's ticket.
2. Discuss the meal with the expeditor or the culinary team member responsible for handling the preparation of the food.
3. If the item takes additional time, inform your team to wait until the special meal is prepared before starting any additional items. An important aspect of food preparation is timing. This will ensure that all the meals are completed at the same time and the family can eat together. I have heard stories of a food allergic guest waiting a long time for their meal, while everyone else in the party has eaten.
4. Remember to check the preparation procedure for potential cross-contact.
5. Wash hands and change gloves before handling the food(s).
6. Prepare the food in the "food allergen safety zone" as directed by the chef, manager, or person in charge.
7. Serve food on the designated plate and place in an area away from other prepared meals.
8. Place the ticket with the special meal.
9. Inform the server the meal is prepared. Either the chef, manager, or person in charge should deliver the food and confirm the order with the guest.
10. The food allergy ticket should be saved for 30 days so if the guest gets sick after they leave your restaurant, you will have documentation of the conversation and what foods were prepared and served to the guest.

Also see Figure 7.7.

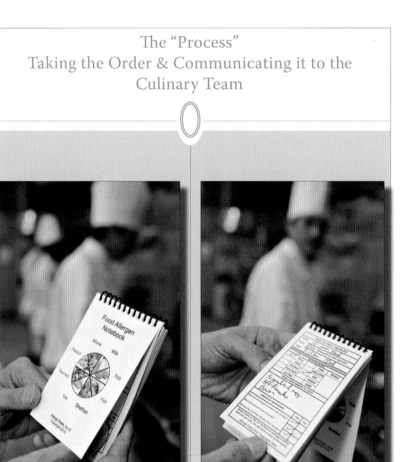

FIGURE 7.6

THE "PROCESS": TAKING THE ORDER & COMMUNICATING IT TO THE CULINARY TEAM.

Food Allergen Safety Process

Guest notifies server of their food allergy or special dietary request

Server REFERS guest to manager, chef or person-in-charge

Person-in-charge REVIEWS dietary request with guest and documents information in the food allergen notebook

Person-in-charge discusses order with chef

Chef REMEMBERS to check ingredients and cross-contact issues for the suggested menu item(s)

Person-in-charge RESPONDS back to the guest to confirm order

Ticket is rung into kitchen. Food allergen checklist sheet is attached to order ticket

Chef or specially trained cook prepares the foods

• Hands are washed and gloves are worn to prepare food
• Food is prepared in FOOD ALLERGEN SAFETY ZONE using specialty tools and equipment
• Food is placed on special plate and put in designated area for pick-up

Food is delivered to guest by the person-in-charge and the order is confirmed with the guest

Manager or chef returns to the table to ensure the guest is satisfied with their meal

FIGURE 7.7

FOOD ALLERGEN SAFETY PROCESS.

STEP 4: RESPOND TO THE GUEST AND INFORM THEM OF YOUR FINDINGS

For the chef, manager, or person in charge, this step may seem out of place since the food has already been ordered and delivered. By now you have already responded to the guest during your visit to the table and would have covered any issues that the guest may have had. What should be done next is to follow-up with the guest in a few minutes to see if they are satisfied with the meal.

Following the 4 R's is simple and will be an asset to your operation. Now that you are focused on cross-contact as well as cross-contamination, you will become more familiar with your menu items and kitchen operations. You will find it easier to suggest menu options for guests with similar food allergies and start realizing that you can create safe, great tasting food and lasting memories for your guests with food allergies.

CHAPTER REVIEW

Food allergen safety should be added to your list of important tasks you undertake daily. Daily communication with your team about the importance of food allergen safety and how the procedure works will keep everyone prepared when you receive the next food allergy request.

Establishing a HACCP program for food allergen safety can be time consuming, but it is essential in developing a sustainable food allergen safety program. Purchase the necessary equipment and specialty products, and have them placed in their designated area. Keep your recipes updated with current ingredient changes or substitutions, and make sure that this is properly communicated to your servers and cooks. Communicate the correct information to guests and let them make the final decision on what they will eat. Keep it simple, fresh, and safe. This is the easiest way to keep your guests safe, happy, and loyal customers for years to come.

ENDNOTES

1. U.S. Food and Drug Administration (FDA), "Hazard Analysis & Critical Control Points (HACCP)," http://www.fda.gov/Food/FoodSafety/Hazard-AnalysisCriticalControlPointsHACCP/default.htm
2. R. M. Goodrich, K. R. Schneider, and R. H. Schmidt, "HACCP: An Overview," August 2005. http://edis.ifas.ufl.edu/pdff.les/FS/FS122200.pdf
3. U.S. Food and Drug Administration (FDA), "Chapter 3—Developing Your Food Safety System for Managing Food Safety: A Manual for the Voluntary Use of HACCP Principles for Operators of Food Service and Retail Establishments," http://www.fda.gov/Food/FoodSafety/Retail-FoodProtection/ManagingFoodSafetyHACCPPrinciples/Operators/ucm078002.htm

4. FDA, "Chapter 3."
5. Ibid.
6. Ibid.
7. American Latex Allergy Association, "Latex Cross-Reactive Foods Fact Sheet," http://www.latexallergyresources.org/News/newsArticle.cfm?ArticleID=95; http://digestive.niddk.nih.gov/ddiseases/pubs/lactose-intolerance/Lactose_Intolerance.pdf
8. Ibid.
9. FDA, "Chapter 3."
10. Ibid.
11. Ibid.

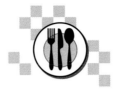

CHAPTER 8

Menu Creation

Auguste Escoffier, "The Chef of Kings and The King of Chefs," was the father of today's modern cuisine and way ahead of his time. His greatest accomplishment was to simplify the overextravagant meals of his predecessors. One of his famous sayings was "Above all, keep it simple." This is my philosophy when it comes to cooking for people with food allergies. My motto is "Keep the food simple to keep the guest safe."

One way to accomplish this is by using special dietary products (SPDs) made specifically for this purpose. Special dietary products will make it easier for you to meet many food allergy and special dietary requests while preparing the foods using safe ingredients. Without the use of SDPs, multiply food allergies and some special diets will be hard to accommodate with what is on a standard restaurant menu.

Increased awareness of food allergies, food intolerances, and special diets has inspired many entrepreneurs to start companies that prepare a variety of products that meet this growing market. Even large companies like King Arthur Flour, General Mills, Rich's, Kellogg's, and Cargill are starting to expand their product offerings to include gluten-free mixes, breads, and desserts that are very good and easy to use.

In this chapter we will review some of the special dietary products I have used. I have provided sample menus utilizing these products that will meet a variety of food allergies and special diets.

IN THE TEST KITCHEN

I have had the opportunity to test many products over the years. It is my hope that this experience will save you time in finding the right products for your operation. When I started experimenting with special dietary products, I had to retrain myself to think differently about these products. First, I had to realize that these products would not behave in the same way their mainstream counterparts would. Second, they would not have the same flavor profiles. Third, regardless of what I thought it tasted like, the product would probably taste good to a guest that has been eating this type of food and had never eaten something like this in a restaurant.

An example of this was trying to melt cheese alternatives. Many of them would not melt or blend into sauces, and the taste—well there were some that I just had to spit out. Gluten-free breads were another one of those exciting taste adventures. Many types of bread would just crumble when they thawed or would be dry within minutes of sitting in the open air. I tested many products until I decided on the ones that would meet our requirements. My goal was to have the best product that was easy to use, easy to obtain, and tasted as close to its counterpart as possible. Luckily for you, today new special dietary products are quickly entering the market and are of higher quality than their predecessors.

If you decide to test your own products, here are the six criteria I used to evaluate each one.

1. The product must meet multiple food allergies: wheat/gluten, milk, eggs, peanuts, and tree nuts. This would allow the product to be served to as many guests as possible without having to carry a large inventory of specialty products.
2. The product must taste good and should have similar flavor profiles to the mainstream item it represents.
3. The product is individually packed or is packed in small quantities.
4. The product is either shelf-stable or could be frozen.
5. It is possible to obtain ingredient and product statements from each company.
6. The product should be easily attainable from either a vendor or local grocery store.

These steps should help you sort through many products right away. It is important to mention that not all of the products in this chapter meet the first criterion. I choose these items because they were excellent products and met a specific meal period or were highly requested by guests.

Real Life Experience: Got Any Packaged Foods?

Prepackaged foods are wonderful. It's not wasteful to open a new container of sorbet for the milk allergic guest or a new container of Earth Balance Naturally Buttery Spread so a child can have something safe to spread on his corn or baked potato. A trip to the emergency room is much more expensive. Allergy-friendly ice "creams," sorbets, cookies, granola bars, pretzels, and tortilla chips can really make a food allergic guest's day. Unlike your regular guests, those with food allergies (celiac disease or those on a GFCF [gluten-free casein-free] diet) love to be served foods that are in the wrapper because serving food is one more way for cross-contact to occur.

Gina Clowes

FIGURE 8.1

SPECIAL DIETARY PRODUCT SHEET.

Manufacturer	Products	Allergen Information	Manufacturing Information
AllergyFree Foods 310 West Hightower Drive Dawsonville, GA, USA 30534 Phone: 706-265-1317 Fax: 706-265-1281 E-mail: info@allergyfreefoods.com www.allergyfreefoods.com	**Chef Joel's Recommendations:** Pancake, All-purpose Muffin, Pizza Crust mixes, breaded chicken nuggets, tenderloins and breasts. **Available in food service packs.	Free of gluten, wheat, milk, eggs, peanuts, tree nuts, fish, shellfish, soy, and corn.	Dry mixes are produced in a dedicated allergen-free facility. Breaded chicken products are produced in a facility with strict Good Manufacturing Practices (GMPs) in place to prevent cross-contact. All products are tested by Silliker® Food Safety & Quality Solutions.
Amy's Kitchen Inc. Box 449 Petaluma, CA, USA 94953 Phone: 707-578-7270 Fax: 707-578-7995 E-mail: amy@amyskitchen.com www.amyskitchen.com	**Chef Joel's Recommendations:** Rice Mac & Cheese, Single Serve Rice Crust Roasted Vegetable Pizza, Baked Ziti Bowl	Amy's makes over 75 products that are gluten-free and others are dairy (milk) free. No meat, shellfish, poultry, eggs, or peanuts are used in their products.	Gluten-free products made in a shared facility with strict GMPs in place to prevent cross-contact.

Company	Products	Allergen Info	Notes
The Birkett Mills 163 Main Street Penn Yan, NY, USA 14527 Phone: 315-536-3311 Fax: 315-536-6740 E-mail: custserv@thebirkettmills.com www.thebirkettmills.com	Pocono (cream of buckwheat, buckwheat groats, buckwheat flour, Kasha), Larrowe (instant buckwheat pancake mix).	Gluten-free.	Dedicated facility that only produces buckwheat. Products are randomly tested for gluten.
Bob's Red Mill Natural Foods Inc. 13521 SE Pheasant Court Milwaukie, OR, USA 97222 Phone: 800-553-2258 or 503-654-3215 Fax: 503-653-1339 www.bobsredmill.com	**Chef Joel's Recommendations:** GF/DF All-purpose Baking, Brownie, and Pancake mixes.	Specialty mixes are gluten, wheat, and dairy (milk) free.	Dedicated gluten-free production facility with their own laboratory to test for gluten in their products.

continued

Disclaimer: Allergen information listed is based on current information from package labels or company website. The products may or may not be free of other common allergens or a food allergen ingredient may be used to prepare the product. Contact manufacturer for additional information or visit their website for the most current allergen information. Always read ingredient labels to ensure a food allergen is not present before preparing and serving a guest.

FIGURE 8.1 (CONTINUED)
SPECIAL DIETARY PRODUCT SHEET.

Manufacturer	Products	Allergen Information	Manufacturing Information
Cherrybrook Kitchen, Inc. 20 Mall Road Burlington, MA, USA 01803 Phone: 866-458-8225 or 781-272-0400 Fax: 781-272-4460 E-mail: info@cherrybrookkitchen.com www.cherrybrookkitchen.com	Dry mixes for cookies, cakes, brownies, pancakes and premade frostings.	All mixes are free of milk, eggs, peanuts, and tree nuts and other products are gluten-free.	Equipment is thoroughly cleaned and tested for cross-contact. Products are tested for peanuts, milk, egg, and gluten.
Cuisine Santé, HACO Ltd., CH-3073 Guemligen, Switzerland USA Distributor: Swiss Chalet Fine Foods 9455 NW-40 Street Road Miami, FL, USA 33178 Phone: 305-592-0008 Fax: 305-702-5395 E-mail order: order@scff.com www.scff.com	**Chef Joel's Recommendations:** Flavored stock mixes—beef, chicken and vegetable; Demi-Glace Brown Sauce mix; and White Roux/Roux Blanc mix. **Only available in food service packs.	Cuisine Santé is a line of dehydrated mixes that are free of gluten, wheat, dairy (milk), casein, eggs, nuts, soy, MSG, hydrogenated fats, and trans fats. Products are vegan.	Products made in a shared facility and every batch is tested for gluten. Certified by GFCO.

	Chef Joel's Recommendations:	All products free of
Divvies, LLC Made to Share Oakridge Common South Salem, NY, USA 10590 Phone: 914-533-0333 E-mail: madetoshare@divvies.com www.divvies.com	**Chef Joel's Recommendations:** Individually packaged cookies, cupcakes, chocolate chips, candies, and popcorn.	All products free of milk, eggs, peanuts, and tree nuts.	Divvies cookies, popcorn and cupcakes are made in a dedicated facility and their ingredients are certified allergen-free. They conduct routine testing to minimize the risk of cross-contact.
Earth Balance™ 7102 LaVista Place, Suite 200 Longmont, CO, USA 80503 Phone: 201-421-3970 Fax: 201-568-6374 www.smartbalance.com www.earthbalancenatural.com	**Chef Joel's Recommendations:** Earth Balance Natural Buttery Spread, Soy-Free and soymilk.	All Earth Balance products are free of milk/casein/lactose, eggs, peanuts, gluten, cholesterol and genetically modified organisms (GMOs).	Contact company for current manufacturing practices.

continued

Disclaimer: Allergen information listed is based on current information from package labels or company website. The products may or may not be free of other common allergens or a food allergen ingredient may be used to prepare the product. Contact manufacturer for additional information or visit their website for the most current allergen information. Always read ingredient labels to ensure a food allergen is not present before preparing and serving a guest.

FIGURE 8.1 (CONTINUED)
SPECIAL DIETARY PRODUCT SHEET.

Manufacturer	Products	Allergen Information	Manufacturing Information
Eco-Cuisine, Inc. A Flexitarian® True to Nature Company P.O. Box 17878 Boulder, CO, USA 80308 Phone: 303-402-0289 Fax: 303-402-0246 E-mail: ron@eco-cuisine.com www.ecocuisine.com	Vegetarian and vegan dry mixes for puddings, frostings, and pie fillings. **Available in food service packs.	All products free of milk, eggs, peanuts, tree nuts, fish, and shellfish.	Product made in a shared facility but is free of tree nuts. They follow strict GMPs to prevent cross-contact.
Ener-G Foods 5960 1st Avenue South Seattle, WA, USA 98108 Phone: 800-331-5222 or 206-767-6660 Fax: 206-764-3398 customerservice@ener-g.com www.ener-g.com	**Chef Joel's Recommendations:** Tapioca dinner rolls, hamburger and hotdog buns, light brown-rice loaf, and egg replacer.	Products are free of major food allergens, sesame, and corn, and some are low-protein and vegan.	Dedicated gluten-free, dairy-free facility and kosher certified facility.

Enjoy Life Natural Brands 3810 N. River Road Schiller Park, IL, USA 60176 Phone: 888-503-6569 or 847-260-0300 Fax: 847-260-0306 Info@enjoylifefoods.com www.enjoylifefoods.com	Cereal, granola, bagels, chocolate chips, individually wrapped cookies, chocolate bars, and snack bars.	Products free of the top food allergens including corn and potato.	Manufactured in a dedicated allergen-free facility. Certified kosher facility and products certified by GFCO.
French Meadow Bakery™ A RICH'S® Company 1000 Apollo Road Eagan, MN, USA 55123 Phone: 651-286-7861 or 1-877-No-Yeast Fax: 651-454-3327 www.frenchmeadow.com	**Chef Joel's Recommendations:** Fudge brownie, Chocolate Chip cookie (both individually wrapped), par-baked pizza crust, and Italian rolls. **Available in food service packs.	Products are free of milk/casein/lactose, peanuts and gluten.	Manufactured in a dedicated gluten-free facility. Gluten-free products are certified by GFCO.

continued

Disclaimer: Allergen information listed is based on current information from package labels or company website. The products may or may not be free of other common allergens or a food allergen ingredient may be used to prepare the product. Contact manufacturer for additional information or visit their website for the most current allergen information. Always read ingredient labels to ensure a food allergen is not present before preparing and serving a guest.

FIGURE 8.1 (CONTINUED)
SPECIAL DIETARY PRODUCT SHEET.

Manufacturer	Products	Allergen Information	Manufacturing Information
Garden Protein International 200-12751 Vulcan Way Richmond, BC, Canada V6V 3C8 Phone: 1-877-305-6777 or 604- 278-7300 Fax: 604-278-8238 www.gardein.com	**Chef Joel's Recommendations:** Chick'n Filet in a Tuscan Tomato Marinade, Chick'n Satay in a Chili Lime Marinade, Beef less Burger, and Chick'n Strips. **Available in food service packs.	Products are meat-, egg-, and dairy-free.	Produced in a shared facility that makes soy and wheat products. Facility is peanut-free.
Kettle Cuisine 270 Second Street Chelsea, MA, USA 02150 Phone: 877-302-7687 or 617-884-1219 Fax: 617-884-1041 E-mail: contactus@kettlecuisine.com www.kettlecuisine.com	Prepares a variety of gluten-free frozen soups (single-serve, microwavable). **Only available in food service packs.	Gluten-free.	GF soups are made under strict GMPs to prevent cross-contact and each batch is tested for gluten. Gluten-free products are certified by GFCO.

Company	Chef Joel's Recommendations	Notes
Kinnikinnick Foods 1.940-120 Street Edmonton, AB, Canada t5h 3p7 Phone: 877-503-4466 or 780-424-2900 Fax: 780-421-0456 E-mail: info@kinnikinnick.com www.kinnikinnick.com	**Chef Joel's Recommendations:** Bagels, donuts, muffins, and waffles.	All products are free of gluten, wheat, and milk/casein/lactose except for cheese bread.	Dedicated gluten- and nut-free facility. On-site quality control lab that tests for gluten using the highly sensitive ELISA test.
Namaste Foods, LLC P.O. Box 3133 Coeur d' Alene, ID, USA 83816 Phone: 866-258-9493 or 208-772-6325 Fax: 208-772-4318 E-mail: admin@namastefoods.com www.namastefoods.com	**Chef Joel's Recommendations:** Chocolate, vanilla, and spice cake mix. **Available in food service packs.	Products are free of milk/casein/lactose, peanuts, tree nuts, soy, gluten, wheat, corn, and potato.	Made in a dedicated facility free of gluten, wheat, soy, corn, potato, peanuts, tree nuts, dairy, and casein.

continued

Disclaimer: Allergen information listed is based on current information from package labels or company website. The products may or may not be free of other common allergens or a food allergen ingredient may be used to prepare the product. Contact manufacturer for additional information or visit their website for the most current allergen information. Always read ingredient labels to ensure a food allergen is not present before preparing and serving a guest.

FIGURE 8.1 (CONTINUED)
SPECIAL DIETARY PRODUCT SHEET.

Manufacturer	Products	Allergen Information	Manufacturing Information
Nature's Path Foods Inc. 9100 Van Horne Way Richmond, BC, Canada v6x 1w3 Phone: 888-808-9505 or 604-248-8777 E-mail: consumer_services@ naturespath.com www.naturespath.com	**Chef Joel's Recommendations:** EnviroKidz snack bars, Organic Home-style Waffles and cereals. **Available in food service packs.	Gluten-free.	Produced in a facility that uses peanuts, tree nuts and milk. They follow strict GMPs to prevent cross-contact. Gluten-free products are certified by GFCO.
Nonuttin' Foods, Inc. P.O. Box 204 Duncan, BC, Canada v9l 3x3 Phone: 866-714-5411 or 250-175-1481 Fax: 306-542-3951 Email: info@nonuttin.com www.nonuttin.com	Manufacturers of trail mix, baking ingredients, granola bars, and snacks made with pure, uncontaminated oats.	Products are free of milk, eggs, peanuts, tree nuts, sulfites, preservatives, color, and artificial flavors.	Dedicated gluten-free facility.

	Chef Joel's Recommendations:	Many of the products	Contact company for current
Rice Dream Taste the Dream Consumer Relations The Hain Celestial Group, Inc. 4600 Sleepytime Drive Boulder, CO, USA 80301 Phone: 800-434-4246 Fax: 303-581-1520 E-mail: consumerrelations@hain-celestial.com www.imaginefoods.com www.tastethedream.com	Original rice milk (shelf-stable 8-ounce containers), Rice Dream non-dairy frozen desserts (organic vanilla).	are free of milk/casein/lactose, eggs, and gluten. Rice products are free of the top eight food allergens.	manufacturing practices.
Silk® White Wave Foods Company Consumer Affairs 12002 Airport Way Broomfield, CO, USA 80021 Phone: 888-820-9283 or 303-635-4000 www.silksoymilk.com www.silksoybeverage.ca	Manufacture soymilk, yogurt and creamers. **Chef Joel's Recommendations:** Order shelf-stable 8.25-ounce containers for best use. **Available in food service packs.	Products are free of milk/casein/lactose, eggs, MSG, and gluten.	Contact company for current manufacturing practices.

continued

Disclaimer: Allergen information listed is based on current information from package labels or company website. The products may or may not be free of other common allergens or a food allergen ingredient may be used to prepare the product. Contact manufacturer for additional information or visit their website for the most current allergen information. Always read ingredient labels to ensure a food allergen is not present before preparing and serving a guest.

FIGURE 8.1 (CONTINUED)
SPECIAL DIETARY PRODUCT SHEET.

Manufacturer	Products	Allergen Information	Manufacturing Information
Tinkyada Food Directions Inc. 1200 Medford Drive, Unit 8 Scarborough, Ontario, Canada, m1b 2x5 Phone: 416-609-0016 Fax: 416-609-1316 E-mail: jojo@tinkyada.com www.tinkyada.com www.ricepasta.com	**Chef Joel's Recommendations:** Best gluten-free pasta on the market. Brown rice pastas: penne, elbow macaroni, and rotini.	Products free of milk, eggs, peanuts, tree nuts, fish, shellfish, soy, and wheat.	Made in a dedicated gluten-free facility.
Tofutti Brands, Inc. 50 Jackson Drive Cranford, NJ, USA 07016 Phone: 908-272-2400 Fax: 908-272-9492 E-mail: info@tofutti.com www.tofutti.com	**Chef Joel's Recommendations:** Better Than Cream Cheese, Sour Supreme, Premium Frozen Desserts; chocolate and vanilla (pints), and soy-cheese slices.	All products are free of milk/casein/lactose and cholesterol.	Contact company for current manufacturing practices.

Udi's Healthy Foods, LLC	Manufacture whole grain and white sandwich bread, pizza crust, bagels, muffins, cinnamon rolls, and granola.	Gluten-free baked goods are also free of milk/casein/lactose, tree nuts, and soy.	Made in a dedicated gluten-free facility. Certified gluten-free by GFCO.
7010 Broadway, #430			
Denver, CO, USA 80211			
Phone: 303-657-6366			
E-mail: glutenfree@udisfood.com			
www.udisglutenfree.com			
Vege USA, LLC	**Chef Joel's Recommendations:** (Vegan) Black Pepper Steak in Black Pepper Sauce, Orange Chicken in Tangy Orange Sauce, Citrus Sparerib Cutlets in Plum Vinegar Sauce, Shrimp with Sweet Chili Sauce. **Available in food service packs.	Products are free of meat, milk, eggs, peanuts, and tree nuts. Some are also free of wheat.	Many of the products contain soy, and are manufactured in a facility that also processes other products containing wheat.
1425 S. Myrtle Ave.			
Monrovia, CA, USA 91016			
Phone: 888-772-8343 or			
626-386-0800			
Fax: 626-386-0900			
www.vegeusa.com			

Disclaimer: Allergen information listed is based on current information from package labels or company website. The products may or may not be free of other common allergens or a food allergen ingredient may be used to prepare the product. Contact manufacturer for additional information or visit their website for the most current allergen information. Always read ingredient labels to ensure a food allergen is not present before preparing and serving a guest.

Note: This is not a complete list of manufacturers that manufacture special dietary products. For a detailed listing of gluten-free and special dietary manufacturers and other helpful resources see Gluten-Free Diet: A Comprehensive Resource Guide by dietitian Shelley Case, RD at www.glutenfreediet.ca.

SAMPLE MENUS

The following menus are designed for table service restaurants (TSRs; Figure 8.2 and Figure 8.3) and quick service restaurants (QSRs; Figure 8.4), and will accommodate dietary requests for the most commonly requested food allergies. Preparing special menus can assist you with:

- Providing consistency in service and menu selections
- Training of team members on safe serving and cooking procedures
- Establishing standards for communicating to guests with special dietary requests
- Utilizing fewer special dietary products for more meals, which can help eliminate spoilage and inventory issues
- Calculating food cost associated of using special dietary products
- Providing safe and nutritious food for guests with special diets

If you plan on establishing special menus for multiple locations, here is a guideline that will make the transition easy for each location and provide them with menu flexibility.

- Each location should have the opportunity to make substitutions to the menu items, which should be approved by your food safety department or special diets manager.
- Each menu should contain a salad, sandwich, chicken, steak, and/or seafood entrée with steamed vegetables, baked sweet/russet potato, whole grain pilaf, fresh fruit, and dessert.

The vegan menu in Figure 8.5 was prepared for the Humane Society Annual Event at Disney's Coronado Springs Resort in Orlando, Florida. We prepared meals for breakfast, lunch, breaks, and dinner for one thousand guests over a three-day period. The products we used were amazing: easy to use, held well in hot boxes and on buffet lines, and tasted great. Many guests that were not on a vegan diet commented on how great the food looked and tasted. Many of these menu items can easily be incorporated into your current menu offerings and may even be good substitutes for some of your current menu offerings.

Sample Menu

Please advise the server of any additional foods allergies. If you have questions about the menu offerings, please speak to a chef or manager.
Package labels available upon request.

Breakfast

Pancakes[1] or Waffles[2] served with Pure Maple Syrup and Fresh Fruit
Gluten-Free Rolled Oats[3] served with Brown Sugar, Raisins and Milk
Scrambled Eggs, Roasted Red Potatoes, Bacon and Fresh Fruit

Lunch

Rice Crust Cheese Pizza[4]
Served with Seasonal Vegetables Sticks and White Bean Dip

Rice Macaroni & Cheese[4]
Served with green salad and fresh fruit

Grilled Cheese Sandwich[5,6]
Served with fresh fruit

Brown Rice Pasta[7] with Fresh Vegetable and Marinara Sauce
Served with fresh fruit and a Tapioca Roll[5]

Seared Hamburger served on a Tapioca Bun[5] with baked French Fries

Dinner

Items served with a choice of steamed or roasted vegetables, baked sweet potato or buckwheat pilaf, fresh fruit and a tapioca roll

Baked Chicken Breast with Cucumber-Corn Relish

Seared Steak with Onion-Raisin Jam

Middle-Eastern Spiced Pork Tenderloin with White Balsamic Fruit Chutney

Salmon En Papillote drizzled with Herb Oil

Additional time is required to prepare these meals.

Product information

[1] AllergyFree Foods
[2] Van's Waffles
[3] Bob's Red Mill
[4] Amy's Products
[5] EnerG Foods
[6] Galaxy Vegan Cheese
[7] Tinkyada Pasta
[8] French Meadow Bakery

Desserts

Quinoa Crepes, Apple Butter, Fresh Fruit

Fudgie Chocolate Brownie,[8] Vanilla Bean Ice Cream, Strawberry Sauce

Giant Chocolate Chip Cookie[8]
Ice Cream Sandwich, Strawberry Sauce, Real Whipped Cream

Rice Dream and Tofutti Frozen Desserts available upon requests

FIGURE 8.2

TABLE SERVICE MENU FOR GUESTS ON A GLUTEN-FREE DIET.

Sample Menu

Please advise the server of any additional foods allergies. If you have questions about the menu offerings, please speak to a chef or manager.
Package labels available upon request.

Breakfast

Pancakes[1] or Waffles[2] served with Pure Maple Syrup and Fresh Fruit
Gluten-Free Rolled Oats[3] or Grits served with Brown Sugar and Soy[4] or Rice Milk[5]
Scrambled Eggs, Roasted Red Potatoes, Bacon and Fresh Fruit

Lunch	Dinner
Items served with Fresh Fruit	*Items served with a choice of steamed or roasted vegetables, baked sweet potato or buckwheat pilaf, fresh fruit and a tapioca roll*
Non-Dairy Rice Crust Cheeze Pizza[6] Served with Seasonal Vegetables Sticks and White Bean Dip	Breaded Chicken Tenderloins[1]
Vegan Rice Macaroni & Cheeze[6] Served with green salad and fresh fruit	Baked Chicken Breast with Cucumber-Corn Relish
Grilled Cheese Sandwich[7,8] Brown Rice Pasta[9] with Fresh Vegetable and Marinara Sauce Served with a Tapioca Roll[7]	Seared Steak with Onion-Raisin Jam
Seared Hamburger served on a Tapioca Bun[7] with baked French Fries	Middle-Eastern Spiced Pork Tenderloin with White Balsamic Fruit Chutney
Breaded Chicken Tenderloins[1] with baked French Fries	Salmon En Papillote drizzled with Herb Oil *Additional time is required to prepare these meals.*

Product information	Desserts
[1] AllergyFree Foods [2] Van's Waffles [3] Bob's Red Mill [4] Silk Soymilk [5] Rice Dream Classic [6] Amy's Products [7] EnerG Foods [8] Galaxy Vegan Cheese [9] Tinkyada Pasta [10] French Meadow Bakery [11] Rice Dream or Tofutti Frozen Dessert	Quinoa Crepes, Apple Butter, Fresh Fruit Fudgie Chocolate Brownie,[10] Vanilla Bean Ice Cream,[11] Strawberry Sauce Giant Chocolate Chip Cookie[10] Ice Cream Sandwich,[11] Strawberry Sauce, Hershey's Chocolate Syrup *The brownie and chocolate chip cookie can be served in the original package, upon request.*

FIGURE 8.3

TABLE SERVICE MENU FOR GUESTS ON A GLUTEN-FREE CASEIN-FREE DIET.

Sample Menu

Please advise the server of any additional foods allergies. If you have questions about the menu offerings, please speak to a chef or manager.
Package labels available upon request.

Breakfast

Items served with fresh fruit

Pancakes[1] or Waffles[2] served with Pure Maple Syrup
No W/G/M/E/S/P/TN added

GF Rolled Oats[3] served with Brown Sugar and Soy[4] or Rice Milk[5]
No W/G/M/E/P/TN added

Scrambled Eggs, Roasted Red Potatoes, Bacon
No W/G/M/S/P/TN added

Lunch & Dinner

Items served with fresh fruit

Non-Dairy Rice Crust Cheeze Pizza[6]
Served with a Tapioca Roll[7]
No W/G/M/E/P/TN added

Vegan Rice Macaroni & Cheeze[6]
Served with a Tapioca Roll[7]
No W/G/M/E/P/TN added

Baked Cheese Sandwich[7,8]
No W/G/M/E/P/TN added

*Items served with baked French fries &
fresh fruit*

Seared Hamburger on a Tapioca Bun[6]
No W/G/M/E/P/TN added

Steamed Hotdog on a Tapioca Bun[6]
No W/G/M/E/P/TN added

Breaded Chicken Nuggets[1]
No W/G/M/E/S/P/TN added

Desserts

Packaged Desserts

Fudgie Chocolate Brownie[9]

Giant Chocolate Chip Cookie[9]

Two Chocolate Chip Cookies[10]

Caramel Popcorn[10]

Frozen desserts are scooped to order

Rice Dream[12] Vanilla or Tofutti[12]

Chocolate or Vanilla Frozen
Desserts*

Hagen Daz Raspberry Sorbet*

FIGURE 8.4
QUICK SERVICE MENU FOR GUESTS ON SPECIAL DIETS.

Product information

¹ AllergyFree Foods
² Van's Waffles
³ Bob's Red Mill
⁴ Silk Soymilk
⁵ Rice Dream Classic
⁶ Amy's Products
⁷ EnerG Foods
⁸ Galaxy Vegan Cheese
⁹ French Meadow Bakery
¹⁰ Divvies
¹¹ Rice Dream Frozen Dessert
¹² Tofutti Frozen Desserts
[*] Refer to package ingredient label

Allergen Key

W–wheat
G–gluten
M–milk, casein, lactose
E–egg
S–soy
P–peanut
TN–tree nut

FIGURE 8.4 (CONTINUED)

Product information

[1] AllergyFree Foods
[2] Van's Waffles
[3] Bob's Red Mill
[4] Silk Soymilk
[5] Rice Dream Classic
[6] Amy's Products
[7] EnerG Foods
[8] Galaxy Vegan Cheese
[9] French Meadow Bakery
[10] Divvies
[11] Rice Dream Frozen Dessert
[12] Tofutti Frozen Desserts
[*] Refer to package ingredient label

Allergen Key

W–wheat
G–gluten
M–milk, casein, lactose
E–egg
S–soy
P–peanut
TN–tree nut

FIGURE 8.4 (CONTINUED)

Roasted Vegetables on Caribou Bread

Grilled Flatbread served with Assorted Tapenades

Kung Pao Chick'n[1] with Steamed Rice

Orange Chick'n[2] Satay

Chick'n Fajitas[2]

Guacamole, Salsa, Soy-Sour Cream,[3] Diced Tomatoes, Onions, Black Olives, Jalapenos, and Flour Tortillas

Miniature Chick'n[2] and Beef[4] Taco Salad in Corn Tortilla Cups

Tuscan Breast of Chick'n[5] with Caramelized Red Onions, Tomato Relish, served with Vegan Breads

Stir-Fried Vegetable and Beef Brochette[6] with Chive-Balsamic Glaze

Sweet & Spicy Rice Noodles with Snow Peas and Water Chestnuts

Coconut Rum Tapioca Pudding with Latin Fruit Salsa

Bread Pudding with Brandied Soy Cream[7]

Vegan Brownies

Chocolate Cake[8]

Assorted Cookies[9]

Please advise the server or the Captain of any additional foods allergies. If you have questions about the menu offerings, please speak to a chef or manager. Package labels available upon request.

---

[1] Vege USA Kung Pao Chick'n
[2] Gardein Protein – Chick'n Strips
[3] Tofutti, Better than Sour Cream
[4] Gardein Protein – Beef Strips
[5] Gardein Protein – Tuscan Breast of Chick'n
[6] Vege USA – Black Pepper Steaks
[7] Silk Vanilla Soy Milk & Better than Sour Cream
[8] Namaste Cake Mix
[9] Gluten Free Kneads Frozen Cookie Dough

FIGURE 8.5

CATERING MENU FOR VEGAN DIETS.

SUGGESTED PRODUCTS FOR
STYLES OF SERVICE

Not every product will work for each style of service. Table service or catering can be more flexible in their food offering because of the variety of foods available to them. Whereas quick service or concierge operations have limited products, cooking equipment, and storage issues to deal with. To help you in determining what types of products to use for your style of service, I have provided suggestions for each one (Figure 8.6).

Here are some suggestions on how to use each category of items.

Dry mixes

- Purchase products in retail packages only. This will allow you to prepare small batches that can be used daily. There will be less of a chance of cross-contact and product quality can be maintained. When using dry mixes, they should be prepared the same way every time. Do not change the recipe to meet a different diet. This could cause a guest to have a food allergy reaction and it will contaminate the equipment you are using to cook the product.

Breads and breakfast items

- Many breads and breakfast items come in four, six, or eight pieces per package and are shelf-stable or can be frozen. You can create assorted breakfast pastry plates by separating the items onto plates, covering them with plastic wrap, labeling them, and placing them in the freezer until needed. One or two plates can be pulled out of the freezer daily and held at room temperature until needed. Then they can be heated in the microwave and served.
- A breadbasket can be prepared by placing an assortment of specialty breads or rolls in foil, labeling them, and placing them in the freezer. The foil will keep the bread from coming in contact with particles in the oven when heated. When you get a bread order the foil package can be placed directly into the oven and heated for 5 to 10 minutes. Then it should be served in the foil with a side of olive oil, herb oil, or white bean dip.

FIGURE 8.6

SPECIALTY PRODUCTS AND EQUIPMENT FOR STYLES OF SERVICE.

Style of Service	Dry Mixes	Individually Packaged Breads & Breakfast Items	Individually Packaged Snacks	Individual Beverages	Products That Can Be Cooked in the Microwave	Equipment
Catering	X	X	X	X	X	• Microwave • Individual cooking pans, pots, and utensils. • Colored plates, lids, or a way to identify special meals. • Separate storage area or tram for specialty products. • Separate hot and cold boxes for transporting special meals.

continued

FIGURE 8.6 (CONTINUED)

SPECIALTY PRODUCTS AND EQUIPMENT FOR STYLES OF SERVICE.

Style of Service	Dry Mixes	Individually Packaged Breads & Breakfast Items	Individually Packaged Snacks	Individual Beverages	Products That Can Be Cooked in the Microwave	Equipment
Concierge		X	X	X	X	• Microwave • Colored plates, lids, or a way to identify special meals.
Room Service	X*	X	X	X	X	• Microwave • Individual cooking pans, pots, and utensils. • Colored plates, lids, or a way to identify special meals. • Separate storage area or tram for specialty products. • Separate hot and cold boxes for transporting special meals.

Quick Service		X	X	X	X	• Microwave • Individual cooking pans, pots, and utensils. • Colored plates, lids, or a way to identify special meals. • Separate storage area or tram for specialty products.
Food Courts/ Fast Casual	X	X	X	X	X	• Microwave • Individual cooking pans, pots, and utensils. • Colored plates, lids, or a way to identify special meals. • Separate storage area or tram for specialty products.

continued

FIGURE 8.6 (CONTINUED)
SPECIALTY PRODUCTS AND EQUIPMENT FOR STYLES OF SERVICE.

Style of Service	Dry Mixes	Individually Packaged Breads & Breakfast Items	Individually Packaged Snacks	Individual Beverages	Products That Can Be Cooked in the Microwave	Equipment
Table Service	X	X	X	X	X	• Microwave • Individual cooking pans, pots, and utensils. • Colored plates, lids, or a way to identify special meals. • Separate storage area or tram for specialty products.

X*: Many room service operations get their food from a central restaurant or have a limited menu because of kitchen restraints. It may be best to use premade items instead of utilizing mixes.

Snacks

- Many snack products are now available in food service quantities. You can utilize them in all styles of service as a quick dessert or can be resold as a grab-and-go snack. Many families will be relieved when you offer them a dessert or snack that is individually packaged. They will feel a sense of security that the product is safe if they can open the package themselves. Sometimes I would give guests an extra snack to take with them. This made them very happy.
- If you choose to resell packaged items, designate a spot and label them as special dietary products. This is a great guest satisfier because they will not have to look at all the different food labels until they find one that fits their special diet.

Soy and rice milk

- It is best to use individual packages of soy or rice milk. These can be purchased from some local vendors or grocery stores. Many of them are shelf-stable and only need refrigeration if you will be serving them cold. Great for retail sales, using with dry mixes, and serving to the guest in the original package.

Frozen meals

- There are so many frozen meal products on the market now that it is hard to decide which one to use. I have had success with Amy's products because they are recognized by guests as safe and delicious. Amy's products do not contain any meat, poultry, shellfish, eggs, or peanuts, and Amy's has a variety of gluten-free and dairy-free options. These products are great because you can microwave them when needed and serve them in the original container, providing a safe meal for the food allergic guest. These products can be purchased from a vendor such as United Natural Foods (UNFI) www.unfi.com/Foodservice.aspx or at a local grocery store.

Now that you have a good idea of what products to buy, how to use them, and who to purchase them from, it is time to get out there and prepare simple food safely for your guests with food allergies and special diets.

POINTS TO REMEMBER

- Before implementing the use of any special dietary products, make sure you have the proper equipment to prepare the food safely.
- Properly train all culinary team members on the preparation, use, and service of the product.
- Communicate to the servers that these menu items will take additional time to prepare, how the products are prepared, and how they should be served.
- During team meetings, demonstrate how the items are prepared and provide samples for your staff. This will allow them the opportunity to ask questions about preparation methods and learn the flavor profiles of each item.

Final Note from Gina Clowes

Food allergic guests are grateful. I have found that most families living with food allergies and special diets express their appreciation with words, gratuities, and thank-you cards. Please know that if, for whatever reason, you have not been thanked for going the extra mile, we do appreciate it. Not only have you kept a child safe from an allergic reaction, you've helped them to a seat at the table, something that's been sorely missing from a lot of allergic children's and their families' lives.

Gina Clowes

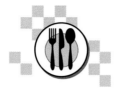

PART III

Abilities

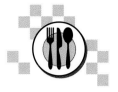

CHAPTER 9

Recipes for the
Professional Kitchen

Serving guests with food allergies is not as hard as it sounds. Your restaurant probably already has menu items that are free from the top eight food allergens. You now need to take the steps listed in Chapter 7 to analyze each recipe to ensure that it is not contaminated with any food allergens during preparation, cooking, and service.

Over the past several years, my wife, Mary, and I have created recipes that eliminate many of the top eight food allergens that are in this chapter. The following recipes are designed to provide you safe and easy ways to prepare menu options that will meet the need of guests with food allergies. Many of the recipes are free of wheat (gluten), milk, peanut, tree nuts, fish, and shellfish. The use of eggs and soy is limited since these ingredients are necessary to create come classic dishes. The recipes yield from one to ten portions, so to reproduce these recipes in larger quantities, follow the steps provided to convert recipes.

RECIPE CONVERSION FORMULA

Working in either the home or professional kitchen, you will be using some form of a conversion formula. You may be increasing an ingredient or having to change a whole recipe depending on how many people RSVP for dinner or at the last minute an event went from 150 to 225 guests. You may be able to do this in your head but to be as accurate as possible, you should use a mathematical equation. The good thing is that these equations can be done with a calculator or a computer recipe program. To convert a recipe you have to calculate the conversion factor of the recipe. Here is the best why to do this:

New Yield/Old Yield = Conversion Factor

Example 1: Increasing a Recipe

Your recipe yields 5 portions and you want to make 15 portions. The following conversion factor will look like this: 15/5 = 3 (conversion factor). Now multiply each ingredient by 3 and the recipe will now yield 15 portions.

Example 2: Reducing a Recipe

Your recipe yields 25 portions and you want to make 10 portions. The following conversions factor will look like this: 10/25 = 0.4 (conversion factor). Now multiply each ingredient by 0.4 and the recipe will now yield 10 portions.

STAPLES FOR THE KITCHEN

OIL AND VINEGAR

Oils and vinegars are essential to any kitchen and are extremely useful in allergen-free cooking. You should have good quality pure oils or a blend of canola and olive oil, which can be used for sautéing, deep fat frying, and salad dressings. Olive oil, balsamic vinegar, and flavored oils can be used as a substitute for premade dressings for salads and can replace butter for bread service. I combine olive oil and canola oil. Many food service vendors offer a blend with different ratios. The benefit in using a blend is that it is less expensive than pure olive oil and you won't have to combine oils to make dressings. I prefer a 60/40 or 70/30 blend, canola to olive oil.

METRIC CONVERSION FACTORS

Weight

- 1 ounce = 28.35 grams
- 1 gram – 0.035 ounces
- 1 pound = 454 grams
- 1 kilogram = 2.2 pounds

Volume

- 1 fluid ounce = 29.57 milliliters
- 1 milliliter = 0.034 ounces
- 1 cup = 237 milliliters
- 1 quart = 946 milliliters
- 1 liter = 33.8 fluid ounces

Temperature

- To convert Fahrenheit to Celsius:
  - Subtract 32. Then multiply by 5/9 (.555).
  - Example: Convert 212°F to Celsius.
    - 212 – 32 = 180
    - 180 × .555 = 100°C
- To convert Celsius to Fahrenheit:
  - Multiply by 9/5 (1.8). Then add 32.
  - Example: Convert 32°C to Fahrenheit.
    - 32 × 1.8 = 57.6 or 58
    - 58 + 32 = 90°F

- Canola oil is made from the canola seed. It contains the lowest levels of saturated fat than any other vegetable oil and is high in monounsaturated fats and has moderate levels of polyunsaturated fats. It is a rich source of vitamin E and is cholesterol-free.
- Olive oil is made from olives. It contains high levels for monounsaturated fat, has moderate levels of polyunsaturated fat, and is a good source of vitamin E and K.
- Extra virgin olive oil comes from the first pressing of unblemished olives done within a day of harvest. No more than 1% of

GARLIC OIL

Yield: 1 quart
Prep time: 5 minutes
Cook time: 5 minutes

There can never be enough garlic oil on hand. I use this garlic oil for everyday cooking, marinating, or just drizzling over grilled meats and vegetables.

Ingredients	Quantity
• Olive oil blend	1 quart
• Fresh garlic cloves, peeled and crushed	12 each
• Kosher salt	¼ teaspoon

Step	Procedure
1	Combine the oil, garlic, and salt in a 2-quart saucepan over medium heat.
2	Heat the oil until the garlic starts to bubble.
3	Simmer on low for 5 minutes.
4	Remove the pan from the heat and let the garlic oil cool before straining the oil into a container.
5	Strain the oil using a chinois or fine mesh strainer into an appropriate container. Reserve the cooked garlic for other uses.
6	Store in the refrigerator until needed.

Allergy note: I have encountered many people with garlic sensitivities. Since garlic is an essential ingredient in the kitchen, people with garlic sensitivities have limited options. You may consider using plain oils instead of garlic or flavored oils for your allergy recipes. Garlic can be added if requested.

HERB OIL

Yield: 1¼ quarts
Prep time: 20 minutes

After 30 years working in various kitchens I have come across some great recipes but there is always one or two that have become part of my repertoire. I love flavored oil and this combination of fresh and dry herbs and spices make flavoring food easy. You will find this savory oil used in many of the recipes in this book. It makes a great marinade for meats, vegetables, and potatoes and can be used to make vinaigrettes and as a dip for bread.

Ingredients	Quantity
• Canola oil	3 cups
• Pure olive oil	2 cups
• Fresh parsley, stems removed	2 ounces
• Fresh rosemary, stems removed	1 ounce
• Fresh garlic cloves, peeled	1 ounce
• Dried thyme	½ ounce
• Kosher salt	½ ounce

Step	Procedure
1	Combine the olive and canola oil in a 2-quart straight-sided container such as a bain-marie or cambro.
2	Add the parsley, rosemary, garlic cloves, dry thyme, and salt to the oil.
3	Using a immersion blender or hand blender, mix the ingredients until smooth. There will be bits and pieces of chopped herbs present in the oil.
4	Store in the refrigerator for up to 2 weeks.

continued

HERB OIL (CONTINUED)

Product tip: The oil should be stirred before each use because the herbs settle to the bottom of the container. I suggest that you experiment with your favorite herbs and spices to create your own blend. You will end up using it in more recipes than you think.

the oil contains oleic acid, which makes the oil taste sharp. Extra virgin olive oil should not be used for cooking.

- Herb oil is made from a blend of canola oil and olive oil, fresh herbs, and garlic. There is always some in my refrigerator to use in cooking, drizzling over grilled foods, making dressings or as a dip. It is an essential part in my allergen-free cooking and is included in many of these recipes.

SPICE MIXES

Spice mixes are a great way to add flavor to food with reducing the possibility of food allergens being added to a dish. Beware of commercial spice mixes; many contain wheat flour or gluten derivatives. I suggest making your own.

MIDDLE-EASTERN SPICE MIX

Yield: 1 cup
Prep time: 5 minutes

While teaching at Kapiolani Community College in Honolulu, Hawaii, I created this recipe for a specialty burger that the students prepared in one of the school's restaurants. The flavors are balanced and add rich color while imparting an aromatic flavor to beef, pork, chicken, and salmon.

Ingredients	Quantity
• Ground cumin	¼ cup
• Ground coriander	¼ cup

continued

MIDDLE-EASTERN SPICE MIX (CONTINUED)

Ingredients	Quantity
• Paprika	¼ cup
• Curry powder	¼ cup
• Kosher salt	2 tablespoons, plus 2 teaspoons

Step	Procedure
1	Whisk together the cumin, coriander, paprika, curry powder, and kosher salt in a mixing bowl.
2	Transfer into an appropriate container and store in a cool, dark place for up to 3 months.

SALT AND WHITE PEPPER MIX

Yield: 1 pound
Prep time: 5 minutes

This is my primary seasoning mix. The white pepper adds an intense peppery taste and blends easily with food without leaving black specs, like black pepper leaves on the food.

Ingredients	Quantity
• Kosher salt	1 pound
• Ground white pepper	½ ounce

Step	Procedure
1	Whisk together the kosher salt and white pepper in a mixing bowl.
2	Transfer the mix into an appropriate container and store until needed.

CHEF JOEL'S ALL-PURPOSE BREADING MIX

Yield: 4 cups
Prep time: 10 minutes

Gluten-free pancake mix can be used in place of making this mix.

Ingredients	Quantity
• Tapioca flour	½ cup (1.8 ounces)
• Cornmeal	½ cup (2.5 ounces)
• Amaranth flour	¼ cup (1 ounce)
• Potato Starch	½ cup (2.4 ounces)
• Sorghum flour	½ cup (2 ounces)

Step	Procedure
1	Combine the ingredients together in a mixing bowl and whisk gently, approximately 1 minute.
2	Store in an airtight container in a cool, dark place for up to 3 months. This mix can also be frozen up to 6 months.

Preparation Tip: Before each use, mix the ingredients to loosen them up. As the mix sits, the potato starch compacts with the other ingredients. This procedure will provide a consistent portioning weight in recipe use.

Standard Breading Procedure

The standard breading procedure is a preliminary preparation for frying and baking. The purpose of this procedure is to provide texture and color to a particular food, protect the food from drying out during cooking, and protect the oil from moisture in the food that will breakdown the oil and shorten its life.

continued

CHEF JOEL'S ALL-PURPOSE BREADING MIX
(CONTINUED)

1. Dry the product first to get a thin, even coating of flour.
2. Season the product or the flour mixture with salt and pepper (step 2). Do not put salt in the breading mix (step 4). The presence of salt in contact with frying oil breaks down the fat and shortens its life.
3. Dip the product in flour mixture (step 2) to coat evenly. Shake off excess.
4. Dip in liquid (step 3) to coat completely. Remove. Let excess drain off so the flour mixture (step 4) will be even.
5. Dip in breading mixture (step 4). Cover with mix and press gently onto the product. Make sure the product is coated completely. Remove. Carefully shake of excess.
6. Fry immediately, or hold for service.
7. To hold for service, place the breaded items in a single layer on a pan lined with parchment paper and refrigerate.
8. Strain the liquid and sift the flour and crumbs as often as necessary to remove lumps.

1	2	3	4	5
Pan to hold product that will be breaded	Specialty flour blend, or pancake mix with salt and white pepper mix	"Liquid" rice or soy milk	"Exterior coating" Chef Joel's All Purpose Breading or pancake mix	Sheet pan, lined with parchment paper for finished product

Safety tip: make sure all strainers are thoroughly cleaned and sanitized before straining allergen-free ingredients. Always refer to food labels or ingredient statements for accurate food allergen information.

SCRATCH STOCKS

Stocks are another staple in the professional kitchen and are essential in the production of sauces, soups, stews, braised items, and sauté dishes. I prefer making stock from scratch, but many food service operations do not have the time, talent, or space to produce scratch stocks. Today you will find many stocks and soup bases available from your local distributor, but beware, many of them contain some of the top eight food allergens, especially wheat, soy, and milk. If you are using stock bases, read the labels to see what food allergens are present. You can also contact your vendor to see if they have any "clean" bases available. Many premier bases only contain meat, vegetables, and seasonings. They may cost more, but are well worth the flavor and piece of mind.

STOCK TYPES, INGREDIENTS, AND PROCEDURES

Stocks are made from bones, vegetables, and seasonings, and sometimes flavored with an acid or wine. Each ingredient must be properly handled to achieve a quality stock. The bones and vegetables should be washed and properly trimmed if needed.

There are five basic stocks:

1. *White stock* can be made from chicken, veal, or beef bones; vegetables; and seasonings.
2. *Brown stock* can be made from chicken, veal, beef, or game bones; vegetables; and seasonings. The bones and vegetables are caramelized before adding the water.
3. *Fish stock or fumet* is made from fish bones or crustacean shells, vegetables, seasoning, and wine. I will not be covering this recipe, since it includes two of the top eight food allergens.
4. *Vegetable stock* is not made with bones. It is made strictly from vegetables such as mirepoix (onions, carrots, celery), leeks, garlic, fennel, turnips, and tomatoes. White wine and seasoning can be added to enhance the flavor and add unique flavors to the finished stock.
5. *Court bouillon* is a simmered liquid with vegetables; seasonings; water; and an acidic liquid, such as lemon or lime juice, vinegar, or wine. It is used for poaching fish and vegetables.

Cooking times: Stock should always be simmered to help clarify the stock and keep the flavors from becoming bitter and off-tasting.

- Beef and veal stock: 6 to 8 hours
- Chicken stock: 3 to 4 hours
- Fish stock: 30 to 45 minutes
- Vegetable stock: 45 to 60 minutes

Mirepoix is a classic vegetable mixture that is used in the preparation of stocks, sauces, and other dishes that need the delicate blend of flavors from the three vegetables (onions, carrots, celery). It is important to know the ratio of this mixture to balance the flavors and aroma of a stock or sauce.

Ratio for 1 pound of mirepoix:

- 8 ounces yellow, sweet, or white onions, first layers of skin removed, chopped in 1–2 inch pieces
- 4 ounces carrots, washed, leaves or stems removed and chopped in 1–2 inch pieces
- 4 ounces of celery, washed, leaves removed and chopped in 1–2 inch pieces

Bouquet garni is another classic herb/seasoning mixture that is used in the preparation of stocks and sauces. It can contain parsley stems, bay leaves, fresh or dry thyme, black peppercorns, cloves and garlic. These ingredients are usually tied in cheesecloth and are called a sachet. The sachet can then be placed in the stock once it is simmering. Once the stock is finished cooking the sachet can be easily removed and discarded.

A bouquet garni consists of the following:

1 bay leaf
¼ teaspoon dry thyme or 5 sprigs of fresh thyme
¼ teaspoon of black peppercorns
6–8 parsley stems
2 whole cloves (optional)
1 garlic clove (optional)

THE SEVEN STEPS TO MAKING A STOCK

There are seven key steps in the preparation of a stock that should also be followed:

1. *Start the stock in cold water.* As the water heats up, it extracts impurities from the bones that will float to the top and are easily removed.
2. *Simmer the stock gently.* This prevents the stock from becoming cloudy so the finished product will be clear.
3. *Skim the stock frequently.* This is a very important step. If the impurities are not removed from the stock, they will eventually be mixed back into the stock and will cause the stock to become cloudy.
4. *Strain the stock carefully.* This process also prevents the stock from becoming cloudy and keeps bone and vegetable pieces from ending up in the stock.
5. *Cool the stock quickly.* The stock should be placed in heat-resistant bags, sealed and placed in an ice bath to help cool the stock quickly.
6. *Store the stock properly.* Properly label, date, and refrigerate the stock to prevent it from spoiling.
7. *Degrease the stock.* Before you use the stock for the first time, remove any fat from the top of the stock. As the stock fully cools, fat droplets will rise to the top, taking participles with them. This should be removed so it does not get into your finished product.

BROWN STOCK

Yield: 1 gallon
Prep time: 10 minutes
Cook time: 3–4 hours for small batches, 6–8 hours for large batches

Since the cooking time is so long for the amount of liquid, add 1 to 2 cups of water halfway through the cooking process to yield 1 gallon of stock.

Ingredients	Quantity
• Water	1¼ gallons

continued

BROWN STOCK (CONTINUED)

Ingredients	Quantity
• Beef, veal, or pork bones, browned	5 pounds
• Mirepoix (carrots, onions, celery)	1 pound
• Bouquet garni sachet	1 each
• Tomato paste	4 ounces

Step	Procedure
1	Prepare the ingredients as directed in the stock section.
2	If the bones are big, cut them into 3-inch pieces and do not wash.
3	Coat the bones with a little canola oil, place in a roasting pan, and place in a 400°F oven until they are brown. Every 30 minutes check the bones and mix them around to brown evenly.
4	Remove the bones from the pan and place in a stockpot, cover with cold water, and bring to a boil. Reduce to a simmer and skim the stock.
5	Remove the excess fat from the pan and toss with the vegetables. Deglaze the pan with water, removing the brown particles. Add this liquid to the stockpot.
6	Place the vegetables in another roasting pan and brown in the oven, making sure the vegetables do not burn. When browned, add to stockpot.
7	Add the bouquet garni and tomato paste; cook for the recommended time.
8	When the stock is done, strain through a china cap lined with cheesecloth, and chill following HACCP guidelines.

COURT BOUILLON (POACHING LIQUID)

Yield: 1 gallon
Prep time: 10 minutes
Cook time: 20 minutes

This liquid can be used for poaching or simmering fresh vegetables for guests with food allergies. The poaching liquid will add flavor to the vegetables without the product coming in contact with other food allergens.

Ingredients	Quantity
• Water	2 quarts
• White wine	2 quarts
• Yellow onions, sliced	4 ounces
• Celery, chopped	4 ounces
• Leeks, washed and chopped	4 ounces
• Bouquet garni sachet	1 each
• Salt	1 ounce

Step	Procedure
1	Place all of the ingredients in a stockpot and bring to a boil.
2	Reduce to a simmer; cook for 20 minutes.
3	Strain the liquid through a china cap lined with cheesecloth; cool according to HACCP guidelines.
4	If the liquid is to be used immediately, pour the liquid into a shallow hotel pan, cover, and keep on the stove over low heat until needed.

VEGETABLE STOCK

Yield: 1 gallon
Prep time: 10 minutes
Cook time: 45 minutes

I prefer using vegetable stock in most of my recipes because is meets more of the requirements for special dietary meals. It is allergy friendly, light in flavor and taste, low in fat, and can be used to prepare vegetarian and vegan recipes.

Ingredients	Quantity
• Water	1¼ gallons
• Canola oil	1½ ounces
• Mirepoix (carrots, celery, onions)	2 pounds
• Leeks, white parts only, washed and chopped	8 ounces
• Mushrooms and mushroom trimmings, chopped	4 ounces
• Fresh garlic cloves, peeled and chopped	½ ounce
• Tomatoes, seeds removed and chopped	4 ounces
• Bouquet garni sachet	1 each

Step	Procedure
1	Heat the oil in a 2-gallon stockpot over medium heat.
2	Sweat the mirepoix, leeks, mushrooms, and garlic for 5 minutes to help release their flavors.
3	Add the tomatoes, bouquet garni, and water. Bring to a boil, then reduce to a simmer.
4	Simmer for 45 minutes.
5	Strain the stock through a china cap lined with cheesecloth. Remove the sachet and squeeze out the excess liquid. Cool following HACCP guidelines.

WHITE STOCK (VEAL, CHICKEN, OR TURKEY)

Yield: 1 gallon
Prep time: 15 minutes
Cook time: 3–4 hours

Since the cooking time is so long for the amount of liquid, add 1 to 2 cups of water halfway through the cooking process to yield 1 gallon of stock. To make a lighter colored stock, replace the carrots with parsnips. I prefer a standard mirepoix because I like the flavor the carrots add to the stock.

Ingredients	Quantity
• Water	1¼ gallons
• Veal, chicken, or turkey bones, washed and blanched	5 pounds
• Mirepoix (carrots, celery, onions)	1 pound
• Bouquet garni sachet	1 each

Step	Procedure
1	If the bones are large, cut them into 3-inch pieces rinse with cold water and place in a stockpot, covered with cold water.
2	Bring to a boil and cook for 1 minute. Strain and rinse the bones.
3	Place the blanched bones in a stockpot and cover with cold water; bring to a boil, skim the particles that rise to the top of the stock; reduce to a simmer.
4	Add the mirepoix and bouquet garni; simmer for recommended time.
5	Strain the stock through a china cap, lined with cheesecloth, and chill following HACCP guidelines.

ALL PURPOSE (GRAVY) SAUCE

Yield: 1 gallon
Prep time: 5 minutes
Cook time: 5 minutes

Ingredients	Quantity
• Brown, white, or vegetable stock	1¼ gallon
• HACO-Swiss Cuisine Santé White Roux	1 pound
• Salt and white pepper mix (p. 211)	2 teaspoons

Step	Procedure
1	Pour the stock into a 2-gallon saucepan over high heat; bring to a boil.
2	Whisk in the white roux; boil for 5 minutes, whisking occasionally.
3	Whisk in the salt and white pepper mix and adjust seasoning if necessary.

Safety tip: Keep the gravy hot in a portable steam table or individual soup kettle with designated label for portioning gravy.
Service tip: This gravy can be used as a base for soups and stews.

ROASTED TOMATO SAUCE

Yield: 3 cups
Prep time: 5 minutes
Cook time: 5 minutes

Ingredients	Quantity
• Roasted tomatoes (p. 247)	1 pound
• Herb oil (p. 209)	1/3 cup
• Tomato paste	2 tablespoons
• Salt and white pepper mix (p. 211)	¼ teaspoon

Step	Procedure
1	Combine the tomatoes, oil, paste, and salt and white pepper mix in a small blender or food processor. Blend until the ingredients are smooth.
2	Pour the sauce into a medium saucepan over medium-high heat; bring to a simmer and cook for 5 minutes.
3	Adjust seasoning if needed.

Service tip: This sauce can be served with pasta or used as a pizza sauce.

SOY BÉCHAMEL

Yield:	1 quart
Prep time:	10 minutes
Cook time:	20 minutes
Food allergen:	Soy

What led me to the position as Special Dietary Manager for Walt Disney World® Resort, was a training class I developed titled "A Look at Lactose Intolerance through the Vegetarian Diet." This was one of the recipes I presented. I never thought this recipe would end up in a book.

Ingredients	Quantity
• Unsweetened, plain, or vanilla soy milk	1¼ quarts
• Sweet onions, chopped	2 ounces
• Whole cloves	2 each
• HACO-Swiss Cuisine Santé White Roux	2 ounces
• Salt and white pepper mix (p. 211)	½ teaspoon

Step	Procedure
1	Heat the soymilk, onions, and cloves in a stainless steel saucepan, over medium heat; cook at a low simmer for 10 minutes. Do not let the soymilk get too hot, as it may burn the bottom of the pan or separate.
2	Bring to a rolling boil; whisk in the white roux; simmer for 5 minutes, whisking occasionally.
3	Strain the sauce through a fine chinois strainer into a stainless steel bowl or container.
4	Season with the salt and white pepper mix.

Service tip: This sauce can be used for soups and small sauces just like a regular milk-based béchamel.

SUNBUTTER® SAUCE

Yield:　　2 cups
Prep Time:　10 minutes

This sauce rocks! It is so rich with a spicy finish; you won't want to make another peanut sauce again. Sunbutter® makes a creamy and chunky version.

Ingredients	Quantity
• Sunbutter® (Chunky, Sunflower Seed Spread)	1 cup
	1 teaspoon
• Ground ginger	½ teaspoon
• Kosher salt	1 teaspoon
• Crushed red pepper flakes	4 teaspoon
• Rice wine vinegar	¾ cup
• Rice milk	Toasted sunflower seeds, crushed
• Garnish	red pepper flakes

Step　Procedure

1　Combine the Sunbutter®, ginger, salt, crushed red pepper flakes, and rice vinegar in a bowl; mix with a stiff wire whisk until smooth.

2　Add ¼ cup of the milk and combine slowly.

3　Add the remaining milk and whisk until the sauce is blended.

　The sauce can be garnished with the toasted sunflower seeds and crushed red pepper flakes just before service.

Safety tip: Be sure to check the allergen statement on the toasted sunflower seeds to see if they have been processed in a plant with peanuts and tree nuts. You would need to share this information with the food allergic guest.

BREAKFAST

Many breakfast items contain milk, eggs, tree nuts, wheat, and sometimes soy ingredients. Unless the restaurant uses special dietary mixes or is trained on how to prevent cross-contact, this meal period can be challenging for many people with food allergies and celiac disease. The following recipes offer options to many of the basic breakfast options that are commonly found on today's menus.

Applesauce Pancakes

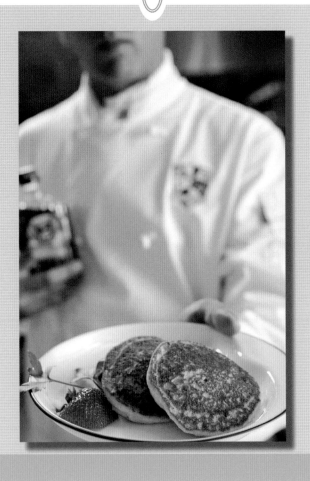

APPLESAUCE PANCAKES

Yield: 2 servings, 3 pancakes each
Prep time: 5 minutes
Cooking time: 5 minutes

Wheat, milk and eggs are essential ingredients in pancakes that give them a light, fluffy texture, and golden color. Over the past several years, I have tasted a variety of specialty pancake mixes, which lack that golden color or light texture.

The key ingredient in pancakes is egg; so finding the best substitute that is readily available in today's professional kitchen was essential. I found unsweetened applesauce is the best substitute. It provides body and helps add color without adding additional sweetness because many specialty pancake mixes have additional sweetener. The best specialty pancake mixes are from AllergyFree Foods, Bob's Red Mill and King Arthur. If you follow the recipe below, you will get 6 to 8 pancakes depending on the mix you use. If you decide to make the whole bag, the batter can be held for one day. You can also prepare all of the pancakes, divide them in packs of 3, wrap them in foil and freeze. The applesauce keeps them moist when reheated. When you get an order, the pancakes can be reheated in the oven, still in the foil.

Ingredients	Quantity
• Pancake mix	1 cup
• Unsweetened applesauce	¼ cup
• Water	⅓ cup
• Canola oil	2 tablespoons

Step	Procedure
1	Preheat a non-stick skillet or griddle over medium-low heat.
2	Combine the pancake mix, applesauce, water and oil in a mixing bowl.

continued

APPLESAUCE PANCAKES (CONTINUED)

Step	Procedure
3	Using a wire whisk, blend the ingredients together to make a slightly lumpy batter. (the applesauce makes the batter lumpy)
4	Lightly grease the cooking surface with canola oil and whip off any excess oil.
5	Using a #24 portion scoop, pour the batter onto the cooking surface.
6	Cook for 1–2 minutes per side.

Note: The batter may be thick, so bubbles may not form around the edges.

Serving suggestions: Serve with Agave nectar or pure maple syrup and Earth Balance® Naturally Butter Spread, Soy-Free.

Safety tip: Cook the pancakes on a designated, non-stick skillet or electric griddle pan using the Allergen Saf-T-Zone™, purple handled spatula from San Jamar.

SWEET POTATO PANCAKES

Yield: 12 pancakes
Prep time: 50 minutes
Cook time: 10 minutes

This recipe was created for the Second Annual Gluten-Free Culinary Summit. The original recipe contained eggs but I have removed them so that these pancakes do not contain the top food allergens.

Ingredients	Quantity
• Gluten-free flour blend	1 cup (4.5 ounces)
• Granulated sugar	2 teaspoons
• Baking powder	2 teaspoons
• Baking soda	½ teaspoon
• Ground flaxseed meal	1 tablespoon
• Warm water	3 tablespoons
• Rice milk	½ cup
• Canola oil	1 tablespoon
• Salt	¼ teaspoon
• Sweet potato; roasted, peeled, and pureed	½ cup

Step	Procedure
1	Preheat a nonstick skillet or griddle over medium-low heat.
2	Sift the flour blend, sugar, baking powder and soda together in a mixing bowl.
3	Combine the flaxseed meal and warm water in another mixing bowl; whisk vigorously until the mixture becomes gelatinous. Let the mixture rest for 2 minutes.

continued

SWEET POTATO PANCAKES (CONTINUED)

Step	Procedure
4	Add the rice milk, oil, and salt to the flaxseed meal; whisk to combine.
5	Add the sweet potato puree to the rice milk mixture; whisk to combine.
6	Add the wet ingredients to the dry ingredients; whisk to combine.
7	Lightly grease the cooking surface with canola oil.
8	Using a #24 portion scoop, portion the batter onto the cooking surface.
9	Cook for 2 minutes per side.

Note: The batter is very thick, so bubbles will not form around the edges.

Carol Fenster's Gluten-Free Flour Blend*

1½ cups sorghum flour
1½ cups potato starch
1 cup tapioca flour or starch

Combine the sorghum flour, potato starch, and tapioca flour in a mixing bowl; slowly whisk until the ingredients are combined. Place in an airtight container and store in a dark, dry, cool location.

---

* 1 cup of a specialty pancake mix can be substituted for the flour blend, sugar, baking powder and baking soda.

BANANA FRENCH TOAST

Yield: 2 servings
Prep time: 10 minutes
Cook time: 3–5 minutes per serving

I learned how to make this from a Disney chef that created many allergen-free breakfast items for his guests. I modified the recipe to work with different types of specialty breads. The batter is sweet enough that the finished product does not require syrup. To make it as allergen-free as possible, use Ener-G Foods, Light Brown Rice Loaf. This bread is more delicate than most gluten-free breads and requires extra care and time to cook. I used French Meadow Bakery sliced gluten-free bread. The bread does contain eggs and soy, so you could use an egg batter with this bread. The batter for the recipe below does not contain the top eight food allergens. The bread will determine what allergens will be in your final recipe.

Ingredients	Quantity
• Sliced bread of choice	4 each
• Banana, ripe	3 ounces
• Rice Dream, Classic Rice Milk	3/4 cup
• Ground cinnamon	1/8 teaspoon
• Granulated sugar	1 teaspoon
• Salt	1/8 teaspoon
• Canola oil (for cooking)	2 tablespoons
• Sliced bananas for garnish	1 each

Step	Procedure
1	Thaw the bread if necessary.
2	Preheat a nonstick flat griddle over medium-high heat.

continued

Banana French Toast

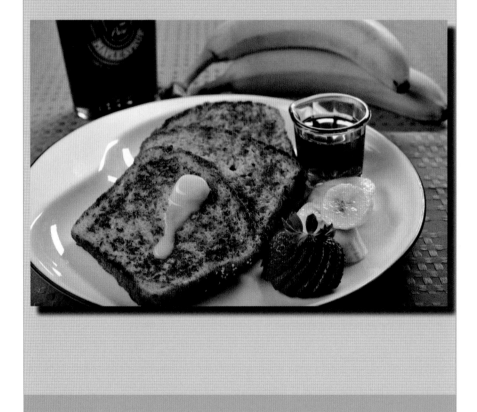

BANANA FRENCH TOAST (CONTINUED)

Step	Procedure
3	Combine the bananas, rice milk, cinnamon, sugar and salt in a blender. Blend until smooth.
4	Pour the batter into a shallow pan, big enough to fit a piece of bread.
5	Place the bread into the batter, one piece at a time, just long enough to coat each side 10–20 seconds. Do not leave the bread in the batter longer or the bread will become soggy and fall apart when removed.
6	Add 1 tablespoon of oil on the griddle and spread around.
7	Place 2 pieces of soaked bread on the griddle and cook for 1 minute.
8	Turn the bread over and cook on the other side until the steam stops rising from the bread.
9	Turn over one more time to brown the other side completely.
10	Serve immediately.

Safety tip: Once you decide on which bread to use, don't change. You must have a designated pan and spatula to prepare the French toast. Do not cook the French toast and pancakes in the same pan if the bread you are using contains a food allergen.
Service tip: Serve with Earth Balance Soy-Free Buttery Spread, pure maple syrup, or Agava nectar and sliced bananas on top.

CHEF JOEL'S BREAKFAST SPECIAL

Yield: Four 6 ounce servings
Prep time: 20 minutes
Cook time: 5–7 minutes
Food Allergens: Eggs, milk

This is a recreation of a recipe I learned while working in an Italian restaurant in Fresno, California. It was our best seller and a great dish for anytime of the day. It is usually finished off with Parmesan cheese and eggs, but it is also good without them.

Ingredients	Quantity
• Canola oil	2 tablespoons
• Fresh garlic, peeled and minced	1 tablespoon
• Yellow or sweet onion, diced	4 ounces
• Ground beef, pork, or chicken	1 pound
• Button or cremini mushrooms, cleaned and sliced	3 ounces
• Frozen chopped spinach, thawed and drained	8 ounces
• Eggs (optional)	2 each
• Parmesan cheese, grated (optional)	1 ounce

Step	Procedure
1	Heat the oil in a large sauté pan over high heat.
2	Add the garlic and onions; cook, stirring often for 1 minute.
3	Add the ground meat; cook, stirring often until the meat is thoroughly cooked. Do not drain the fat.
4	Add the mushrooms; cook until soft.
5	Loosen up the spinach and mix it into the other ingredients. At this point, the dish can be seasoned with salt and served. If you want to add the eggs and cheese, follow steps 6 and 7.

continued

CHEF JOEL'S BREAKFAST SPECIAL (CONTINUED)

Step	Procedure
5	Loosen up the spinach and mix it into the other ingredients. At this point, the dish can be seasoned with salt and served. If you want to add the eggs and cheese, follow steps 6 and 7.
6	Make a hole in the center of the mixture and add 1 tablespoon of oil.
7	Add the eggs; scramble until completely cooked. Sprinkle with the cheese and mix the ingredients together. Serve immediately.

LEMON-CHOCOLATE CHIP SCONES

Yield: 8 each
Prep time: 30 minutes
Cook time: 15 minutes

Oven temperature: 400°F for a conventional oven, 375°F for a convection oven.

The original version of this scone was created for the 1st Annual Gluten-Free Summit, which was held in Copper Mountain, Colorado. Since that summit, we have made changes to the recipe so that it is not only gluten-free, but also free from milk, eggs, peanuts and tree nuts.

Ingredients	Quantity
• Gluten-free flour blend	1¾ cups (6.6 ounces)
• Tapioca flour	½ cup (2 ounces)
• Xanthan gum	½ teaspoon
• Cream of tartar	1½ teaspoons
• Baking soda	¾ teaspoon
• Salt	½ teaspoon

continued

Lemon-Chocolate Chip Scones

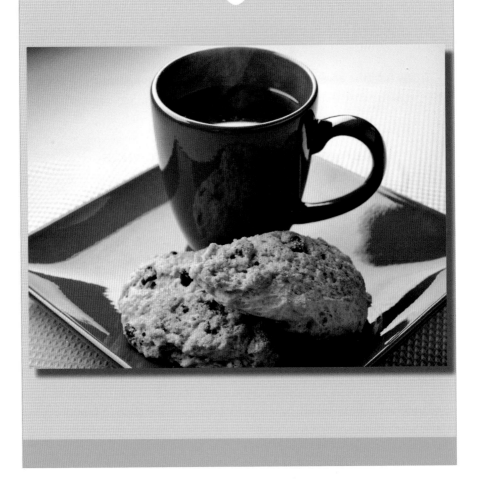

LEMON-CHOCOLATE CHIP SCONES (CONTINUED)

Ingredients	Quantity
• Granulated sugar	2 tablespoons
• Divvies dark chocolate chips*	½ cup (3 ounces)
• Flax meal	1 tablespoon
• Water	3 tablespoons
• Rice milk	⅓ cup
• Lemon	1 each
• Earth Balance Natural Buttery Spread, soy-free, cold	¼ cup (2 ounces)
• Rice milk	⅛ cup
• Cinnamon sugar	1 tablespoon

Step	Procedure
1	Preheat oven to indicated temperature.
2	Sift together the gluten-free flour, tapioca flour, xanthan gum, cream of tartar, baking soda, salt, and sugar in a large mixing bowl. Add the chocolate chips.
3	Whisk together the flax meal and water. Let the mixture sit for a couple of minutes while you zest the lemon. You should have approximately 1 tablespoon of lemon zest. Whisk again the flax meal and water. It will have a gelatinous texture. Add the lemon zest and first rice milk of 1/3 cup to the flax mixture. Whisk gently to combine.
4	Cut the cold Earth Balance natural buttery spread into small pieces and work into the flour mixture with your hands until it resembles a coarse meal.

continued

LEMON-CHOCOLATE CHIP SCONES (CONTINUED)

Step	Procedure
5	Add the rice milk mixture; mix with a rubber spatula by hand just until combined.
6	Using a designated #20 portion scoop, scoop the dough onto a parchment-lined sheet pan. Flatten slightly with a half-cup measure or glass dipped in tapioca flour. Or, for a traditional triangular scone, shape the dough into a 7-inch disc, ¾-inch thick. Using a bench scraper or chef's knife, cut the dough into 8 wedges and set on a prepared baking sheet, spacing them about 2 inches apart.
7	Brush the top surfaces with rice milk. Sprinkle with cinnamon sugar. Bake until golden brown, 12 to 15 minutes; cool the scones on the baking sheet on a wire rack for 5 minutes, then transfer the scones to the rack and cool to room temperature, about 30 minutes. Serve.

Product tip: To make the cinnamon sugar, combine ½ cup granulated sugar with 1 teaspoon of ground cinnamon. Mix well.

Product substitutions: Enjoy Life semi-sweet chocolate chips are dairy-, nut-, and soy-free. Tropical Source semi-sweet chocolate chips are dairy- and gluten-free.

---

* Divvies dark chocolate chips do contain soy lecithin.

CONDIMENTS

Condiments such as chutneys, relishes, and salsas are a great way to make the "center of the plate" ingredient taste exciting, and add color and interest to the plate. Since the majority of these condiments are made from fruits and vegetables, they are a natural alternative for guests with food allergies.

Trio of Dips:
Avocado Smash, White Bean with Roasted Garlic, & Roasted Herb-Tomato

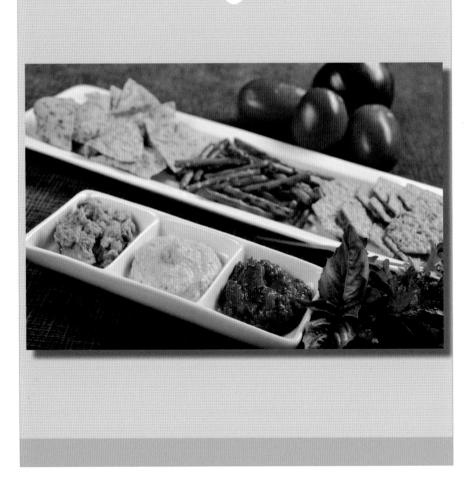

WHITE BEAN DIP

Yield: 2¼ cups
Prep time: 50 minutes
Oven temperature: 400°F

This is my wife's favorite dip. We use it in place of mayonnaise in the Chicken, Grapes, and Tarragon Salad, and have used it in omelets and as a spread for sandwiches.

Ingredients	Quantity
• Great white northern beans, drained and rinsed	2 each, 15 ounce cans
• Garlic cloves, roasted	6 each
• Fresh lemon juice	2 tablespoons
• Fresh parsley, stems removed	2 tablespoons
• Salt and white pepper mix (p. 211)	1 teaspoon
• Extra virgin olive oil	1/3 cup

Step	Procedure
1	To roast the garlic, trim off the top of the garlic bulb to expose the cloves. Brush the top with canola or olive oil and wrap in foil.
2	Bake the garlic in a 400°F oven for 35–45 minutes, or until the garlic bulbs are soft. Set the garlic aside, still in the foil, until cool. (Do not brown the garlic cloves too much. The flavor of brown garlic is too strong for this dip.)
3	Drain and rinse the beans. You may substitute cannellini or white kidney beans for the great white northern beans. The weight of the drained and rinsed beans is 17 ounces.

continued

WHITE BEAN DIP (CONTINUED)

Step	Procedure
4	Squeeze or scoop the roasted garlic flesh from the skins.
5	Process the beans, roasted garlic, lemon juice, parsley, salt and white pepper mix, and oil together in a food processor until smooth. If the dip is too thick, add 2 additional tablespoons of olive oil and process for 30 seconds.
6	Transfer into an appropriate container and refrigerate for up to 3 days.

Variations: To make a lighter version of this dish, use 2 tablespoons of stock or water in place of olive oil. Serve with gluten-free crackers or corn chips and as a dip for vegetables.

AVOCADO SMASH

Yield: 2 cups
Prep Time: 10 minutes

This is a great sandwich spread, dip, or condiment for spicy grilled meats and Mexican food. To retain the "smash" look, smash the ingredients with a fork.

Ingredients	Quantity
• Ripe avocados, seeded and diced	2 each (10 ounces)
• Red onions, minced	1 ounces
• Fresh lemon juice	4 teaspoons
• Fresh cilantro, chopped	1 tablespoon
• Salt and white pepper mix (p. 211)	To taste

Step	Procedure
1	Smash the avocados in a bowl with a fork.
2	Gently fold in the red onions, lemon juice, cilantro, and salt and white pepper mix.
3	Cover with plastic wrap so the plastic wrap is in direct contact with the avocados; refrigerate for 1 hour to blend flavors. Shelf life is 2 days.

BALSAMIC FRUIT CHUTNEY

Yield: 1 quart
Prep time: 35 minutes
Cook time: 20 minutes

The word "chutney" comes from the East Indian word *chatni*. This spicy condiment contains fruit, vinegar, sugar, and spices. It can range in texture from chunky to smooth, and in degrees from mild to hot. Chutney is traditionally served with curried foods but I find it a great accompaniment for grilled meats and many of them are allergen-free.

Ingredients	Quantity
• White or red balsamic vinegar	1 cup
• Apple cider vinegar	1 cup
• White or brown sugar	2 cups
• Canola oil	1 tablespoon
• Sweet onions, diced	4 ounces
• Garlic cloves, minced	2 each
• Granny Smith apples, peeled, cored, and diced	3 cups
• Golden or regular raisins	1 cup
• Ripe banana, peeled and small diced	1 each
• Kiwis, peeled and small diced	3 each
• Strawberries, washed and small diced	3 each
• Fresh mint, minced	1 tablespoon
• Salt and white pepper mix (p. 211)	To taste

Step   Procedure

1   Combine the balsamic, apple cider vinegar, and sugar together in a medium saucepan over high heat; bring to a boil. Reduce to a simmer and cook until the sauce reduces to a syrupy consistency, about 10 minutes.

continued

BALSAMIC FRUIT CHUTNEY (CONTINUED)

Step	Procedure
2	While the vinegars and sugar are cooking, heat the oil in a sauté pan over medium heat; add the onions. Cook, stirring often, until the onions are slightly colored, then add the garlic. Cook for 1 minute.
3	When the vinegar reduction reaches a syrupy consistency, add the apples and onion mixture. Stir to combine; simmer for 10 minutes to soften the apples.
4	Add the raisins; cook for 5 minutes.
5	Remove the pan from the stove and transfer the chutney into a large mixing bowl. Place this bowl into another bowl with ice water (cold water bath). Occasionally stir the mixture to help it quickly cool.
6	When the chutney is cold, add the bananas, strawberries, and kiwis, and stir gently. Do not smash the fruit.
7	Season to taste with salt and white pepper mix.

Variations: To retain the vibrant colors of the fresh fruit, use white balsamic vinegar and white sugar.

RED ONION CHUTNEY

Yield: 10 ounces (Five 2-ounce servings)
Prep time: 10 minutes
Cook time: 20–25 minutes

This condiment can be cooked to order or prepared ahead of time. For best results, keep this chutney warm so the spread does not firm up. This chutney goes best with beef and pork but is also good served with chicken or turkey.

Ingredients	Quantity
• Earth Balance® Natural Buttery Spread, Soy-Free	3 tablespoons
• Canola oil	1 tablespoon
• Red onions, peeled and sliced or diced	1 pound
• Dark raisins or cranberries	2 ounces
• Apple cider vinegar	¼ cup
• Light brown sugar	¼ cup
• Water	¼ cup
• Salt and white pepper mix (p. 211)	¼ teaspoon

Step	Procedure
1	Melt the buttery spread and oil in a sauté pan over medium heat.
2	Add the red onions and sauté for 5 minutes, stirring occasionally so the onions do not burn.
3	Add the dried fruit and sauté for an additional 3 minutes. You may need to add a few tablespoons of water so the ingredients do not burn.
4	Add the apple cider vinegar, brown sugar, and water. Cook until the liquid reduces to a syrup consistency.
5	Remove from the heat and add the remaining 2 tablespoons of buttery spread and mix until melted. Season with salt and white pepper mix.

ROASTED TOMATOES

Yield:	2 pounds
Prep time:	5 minutes
Cook time:	4–6 hours
Oven temperature:	Conventional oven 250°F; convection oven 200°F, low fan setting

This recipe was a favorite of mine while working at Angelica's Café in Honolulu, Hawaii. We used these tomatoes as a garnish for a Walnut-Crusted Goat Cheese and Roasted Tomatoes Salad with Lemon-Thyme Vinaigrette. The tomatoes are so good that I started using them to create different sauces. You will find it in the following recipes: Roasted Tomato Dip (p. 248), Spicy Tomato Vinaigrette (p. 265), and Roasted Tomato Sauce (p. 222).

Ingredients	Quantity
• Roma or plum tomatoes, tops and bottom removed and cut in half through the middle crosswise	5 pounds
• Garlic oil (p. 208)	2 tablespoons
• Fresh garlic cloves, peeled and minced	2 tablespoons
• Salt and white pepper mix (p. 211)	1 teaspoon

Step	Procedure
1	Combine the tomatoes, oil, garlic, and salt and white pepper mix in a mixing bowl; toss to coat the tomatoes.
2	Arrange the tomatoes, cut end sides down, on a sheet pan lined with parchment paper.
3	Slowly bake the tomatoes in the oven for 4 to 6 hours, or until the tomatoes have reduced by half. Check the tomatoes every hour to make sure they are not burning on the bottom of the pan. The finished tomatoes should look slightly shriveled and the bottoms should be slightly caramelized.

continued

ROASTED TOMATOES (CONTINUED)

Step   Procedure

4   Remove the tomatoes from the oven and allow them to cool
         before placing in the refrigerator.

Storage tip: To use as a garnish, arrange them in single rows in a pan. Divide each layer
with parchment paper. This will keep them uniform and in good condition for service.
You can also continue to cook them for 6 to 8 hours to achieve your own oven-dried
tomatoes that are great addition to pasta and salad dishes.

ROASTED TOMATO DIP

Yield: 3 cups (24 ounces)
Prep time: 15 minutes

Ingredients	Quantity
• Roasted tomatoes (p. 247)	1 pound
• Fresh basil, chopped	2 tablespoons
• Fresh parsley, stems removed and chopped	1 teaspoon
• Fresh oregano, stems removed and chopped	1 teaspoon
• Extra virgin olive oil	2 tablespoons
• Salt and white pepper mix (p. 211)	¾ teaspoon

Step   Procedure

1   Combine the tomatoes, basil, parsley, oregano, oil and salt and
         white pepper mix in a food processor and pulse just enough to
         bring the ingredients together.

2   Transfer into an appropriate container. It can be stored in the
         refrigerator for up to 1 week.

Variations: To make a roasted tomato sauce, add 1/3 cup herb oil and 2 tablespoons
tomato paste to the dip; blend in a food processor until smooth.

VINE-RIPENED TOMATO SALSA

Yield: 3 pounds
Prep time: 15 minutes

Salsas are another condiment that is very versatile in today's kitchen. *Salsa* is the Spanish word for "sauce," which can indicate cooked or fresh mixtures. Salsas can range in heat from mild to extremely spicy. Fresh salsas can be covered tightly and refrigerated for up to 5 days while cooked salsas can be held in the refrigerator for 1 month once they are opened.

Ingredients	Quantity
• Yellow tomatoes, vine ripened, seeded and diced	1 pound
• Red tomatoes, vine ripened, seeded and diced	1 pound
• Yellow onions, minced	8 ounces
• Fresh cilantro, chopped	4 tablespoons
• Sweet Thai chili sauce	1 tablespoon
• Rice wine vinegar	4 tablespoons
• Granulated sugar	½ cup
• Salt and white pepper mix (p. 211)	2 teaspoons

Step	Procedure
1	Mix the tomatoes, onions, cilantro, chili sauce, vinegar, sugar, and salt and white pepper mix together in a stainless steel mixing bowl.
2	Cover with plastic wrap and allow the salsa to rest for 1 hour to blend flavors.

Variations: You can substitute any large, fresh tomatoes if yellow ones are not available.

APPETIZERS, SALADS, AND SALAD DRESSINGS

Serving a salad to a guest with food allergies should be an easy process. Unfortunately, it is not. I have heard of many incidents of a food allergy reaction occurring because a server removed an ingredient from a salad and gave it back to the guest without telling them. All food service professionals that handle food allergy requests should remember this saying, "You can always add, but not take away." This applies to all food allergy meal preparations. If you make a mistake, start from scratch.

Vegetable and fruit salads are great options for guest with food allergies. Leave off the eggs, cheese, croutons, nuts, mayonnaise, and cream-based dressings. Using precut fruits and lettuces also helps reduce the rise of cross-contact occurring from improperly washed and sanitized cutting boards, knives, and kitchen sinks used to wash lettuce.

Scratch dressings are a better option because you can control what ingredients are used. Many premade dressings contain food allergens, especially gluten-containing ingredients that do not have to be listed on the ingredient statement per the FDA.

BREADED CHICKEN TENDERLOINS LETTUCE WRAPS

Yield: 4 servings
Prep time: 30 minutes
Cook time: 6 minutes

AllergyFree Foods produces all-natural, allergen-free breaded chicken products that taste just as good as regular chicken tenders. They can be deep-fried, pan-fried, or baked.

Ingredients	Quantity
• AllergyFree Foods, Chicken Tenderloins	16 ounces (1 bag)
• Canola oil, for frying	2 quarts
• Butter or green leaf lettuce	8 leaves
• Avocado Smash (p. 243)	8 ounces
• Vine-ripened tomato salsa (p. 249) or your favorite salsa	8 ounces

Step	Procedure
1	Arrange the lettuce leaves on a round plate or platter.
2	Cook the chicken as directed. Drain on paper towels to absorb excess oil.
3	Slice the cooked tenderloins and arrange them on each lettuce leaf.
4	Top with avocado smash and salsa. Wrap and enjoy!

Safety tip: The chicken tenderloins are best fried and should be fried in a designated fryer, such as a Fry Daddy™ or a tabletop fryer, which can be purchased from your local equipment supply vendor.

Service tip: Lettuce wraps can also be served with sour cream. For guests with milk allergies, soy sour cream can be substituted (the dish would now contain a soy allergen).

Breaded Chicken Tenderloin Lettuce Wraps

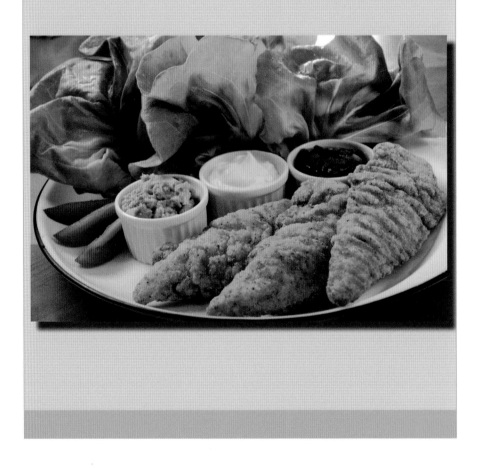

CHICKEN SKEWERS, ROOT VEGETABLE
SLAW, SUNBUTTER® SAUCE

Yield: 9 skewers
Prep time: 10 minutes
Cook time: 10 minutes
Oven temperature: 350°F

I experimented with cutting chicken breasts in different ways to find the best yield, visual appearance, and uses out of one cut. The cubes can be used for skewers, soups and stews, sauté dishes, and salads.

Ingredients	Quantity
• Skinless, boneless chicken breasts, trimmed and cut into 1 ounce cubes	20 ounces
• Herb or garlic oil	2 tablespoons
• Salt and white pepper mix (p. 211)	1/8 teaspoon
• 6-inch wooden skewers, soaked in water overnight	9 each
• Root Vegetable Slaw with Pineapples (p. 260)	1 recipe
• Sunbutter® Sauce (p. 224)	1 recipe

Step	Procedure
1	Mix the chicken cubes, oil, and salt and white pepper mix in a mixing bowl.
2	Cover and marinate in the refrigerator for 2 hours or overnight.
3	Skewer the chicken cubes, three per stick.
4	Preheat a nonstick grill pan or griddle over medium heat; brown the chicken on each side for 1–2 minutes.

continued

Chicken Skewers, Root Vegetable Slaw, Sunbutter® Sauce

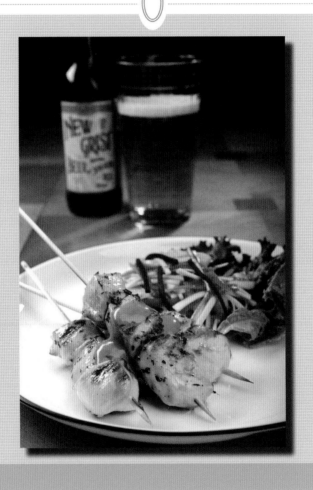

CHICKEN SKEWERS, ROOT VEGETABLE
SLAW, SUNBUTTER® SAUCE (CONTINUED)

Step	Procedure
5	Transfer to a sheet pan lined with parchment paper. If your pan is oven safe, place directly into the oven; bake for 5 minutes.
6	While the chicken is cooking, place 4 ounces of slaw on the allergen-safe plate and portion 2 ounces of sauce into a side dish.
7	When the chicken is finished cooking, place 3 skewers on each plate and serve immediately.

Safety tip: For the skewers, sear the chicken in advance on a designated grill pan and wrap each order in foil. When you get an order, place the chicken, still wrapped in foil, in the oven for 5 to 10 minutes and serve with requested side.

Preparation tip: To prevent the wood skewers from burning, soak them in water for 2 to 4 hours before skewering the chicken.

Equipment tip: The best pan for searing meats is the Cuisinart GreenGourmet® Hard Anodized, 11-inch Square Grill Pan. It has a superior nonstick, heavy duty coating, and is easy to keep clean. It evenly cooks and browns meat with exceptional grill marks.

CHICKEN NUGGET & PINEAPPLE SALAD

Yield: 4–6 servings
Prep time: 15 minutes
Cook time: 10 minutes
Food allergen: Soy

While working as the research and development chef for AllergyFree Foods, Mary and I attended the 4th Annual Gluten-Free Vendor Show. This recipe was created for a cooking demonstration at the show. This recipe is for kids but adults really like it too. I guess there is a little kid in all of us.

Ingredients	Quantity
• AllergyFree Foods Chicken Nuggets	18 pieces
• Shredded lettuce	1 each, 8 ounce bag
• Canned black beans, drained and rinsed	1 each, 15 ounce can
• Vine-Ripened Tomato Salsa (p. 249)	2 cups
• Avocado, pitted and diced	2 each
• Canned pineapple chunks, drained and juice reserved for pineapple glaze	1 each, 20 ounce can

Pineapple Glaze

• Pineapple juice	1 cup
• Brown sugar	1 tablespoon
• Gluten-free Tamari soy sauce (San-J)	1 teaspoon
• Cornstarch or tapioca flour	2 teaspoons

Step	Procedure
1	To prepare the sauce, whisk together the reserved pineapple juice, plus enough water to make 1 cup, brown sugar, soy sauce, and starch in a small saucepan.

continued

CHICKEN NUGGET & PINEAPPLE SALAD
(CONTINUED)

Pineapple Glaze

Step	Procedure
2	Place the pan on the stove over medium-high heat; bring to a boil, whisking occasionally.
3	Boil the liquid for 2 minutes to allow the starch to absorb the liquid and become thick.
4	Remove from the stove and keep warm.
5	Prepare the chicken nuggets based on package directions.
6	While the nuggets are cooking, combine the lettuce, beans, avocado, and pineapple chunks in a mixing bowl; toss ingredients gently.
7	Divide the salad between the plates; top with 2 ounces of salsa.
8	When the chicken is done, remove and place on a paper towel.
9	Arrange 3 nuggets on each salad. Pour 1 ounce of pineapple glaze over each nugget.
10	Serve immediately.

Chicken Nugget & Pineapple Salad

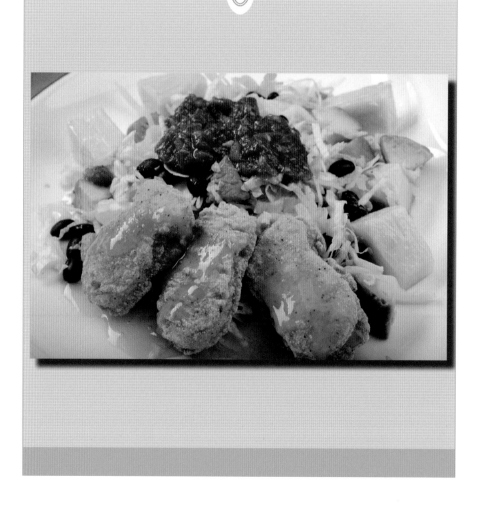

CHICKEN, GRAPES, AND TARRAGON SALAD

Yield: 2 cups
Prep time: 20 minutes
Cook time: 10–15 minutes to cook chicken
Oven temperature: 350°F

The white bean dip is a great substitute for mayonnaise. The flavor is neutral enough to use in other applications where mayonnaise is needed.

Ingredients	Quantity
• Cooked skinless, boneless chicken breasts	12 ounces
• Canola oil	1 teaspoon
• Salt and white pepper mix (pg. 211)	¼ teaspoon and ½ teaspoon
• White Bean Dip (p. 241)	½ cup
• Celery, small diced	half stalk (1 ounce)
• Seedless red grapes, cut in half	1 cup (6 ounces)
• Fresh tarragon, stems removed and chopped	1 tablespoon
• Canned water chestnuts, drained, small diced	¼ cup

Step	Procedure
1	Toss the chicken breasts (approximately 1 pound uncooked) with the oil, and ¼ teaspoon salt and white pepper mix. Arrange chicken on a sheet pan lined with parchment paper.
2	Bake in a preheated 350°F oven for 10 minutes, or until the internal temperature reaches 165°F.
3	Cool the chicken in the refrigerator. When cool, chop the chicken into small pieces.
4	Combine the chicken, white bean dip, celery, grapes, tarragon, and water chestnuts in a mixing bowl; mix thoroughly.
5	Season with the additional ½ teaspoon salt and white pepper mix.

ROOT VEGETABLE SLAW WITH PINEAPPLES

Yield: 8 servings
Prep time: 30 minutes if vegetables are not cut

If you have never tasted raw root vegetables, you are in for a surprise. These vegetables raw add a distinctive taste to any dish and are surprisingly light and refreshing. The slaw is a perfect accompaniment with chicken skewers, grilled meats, or as a sandwich topping.

Ingredients	Quantity
• Daikon radish, peeled and julienne cut	4 ounces
• Carrots, peeled and julienne cut	4 ounces
• Parsnips, peeled and julienne cut	4 ounces
• Beets, peeled and julienne cut	2 ounces
• Pineapple, peeled, cored, and small diced	3 ounces
• Chives, chopped	¼ cup
• Slaw Dressing (pg. 264)	1 cup
• Salt and white pepper mix (pg. 211)	¼ teaspoon

Step	Procedure
1	Prepare the daikon, carrots, parsnips, and pineapple as directed. Combine the ingredients in a mixing bowl with the chives, dressing, and salt and white pepper mix; mix together. Cover and place in the refrigerator.
2	Prepare the beets as directed and place in a bowl of ice water to help "bleed" out the color of the beets. This will help the slaw from getting discolored.
3	Just before service, add the beets; toss and serve.

THREE-BEAN SALAD

Yield: 1 quart
Prep time: 20 minutes
Cook time: 5 minutes to cook the onions

Ingredients	Quantity
• Canned black beans	1 each, 15 ounce can
• Canned Great White Northern beans	1 each, 15 ounce can
• Canned red beans	1 each, 15 ounce can
• Sweet onions, small diced	½ cup
• Canola oil	1 tablespoon
• Red bell peppers, small diced	½ cup
• Green bell peppers, small diced	½ cup
• Champagne Vinaigrette (p. 262)	½ cup
• Salt and white pepper mix (p. 211)	To taste

Step	Procedure
1	Drain and rinse the beans thoroughly. Set aside.
2	Heat the canola oil in a sauté pan over medium heat. Add the onions; cook for 3–5 minutes, stirring occasionally, until the onions are browned.
3	Combine the beans, caramelized onions, bell peppers, champagne vinaigrette, and salt and white pepper mix in mixing bowl; toss to combine the ingredients.
4	Store in a stainless steel container, covered until needed.

Service tip: Check the salad daily. The beans will absorb dressing while it sits overnight and will need more to enhance the flavor.

CHAMPAGNE VINAIGRETTE

Yield: 3 cups
Prep time: 5 minutes

Ingredients	Quantity
• Champagne vinegar	1 cup
• Olive oil	2 cup
• Extra Virgin olive oil	½ cup
• Garlic cloves, chopped	2 tablespoons
• Italian flat parsley, stems removed	4 tablespoons
• Salt and white pepper mix (p. 211)	1 teaspoon

Step	Procedure
1	Combine the vinegar, oils, garlic, and parsley in a blender; blend until the ingredients are emulsified.
2	Season to taste with the salt and white pepper mix.
3	Transfer the vinaigrette into a suitable container and store in the refrigerator until needed.

ROASTED GARLIC–HERB VINAIGRETTE

Yield: 1 quart
Prep time: 5 minutes

Here is a way to incorporate the herb oil and leftover garlic from the garlic oil. Waste not, want not, I always say.

Ingredients	Quantity
• Roasted garlic (or reserved garlic from garlic oil, p. 208)	2 tablespoons 4 teaspoons
• Dry mustard	1 cup
• Balsamic vinegar	3 cups
• Herb oil (p. 209)	1 teaspoon
• Salt and white pepper mix (p. 211)	

Step	Procedure
1	Combine the garlic, mustard, and vinegar in a blender.
2	Blend the ingredients together.
3	While the blender is running, remove the top and slowly pour the herb oil into the mixture. Blend until the ingredients are emulsified.
4	Season with the salt and white pepper mix and blend for 20 seconds.
5	Transfer the vinaigrette into a suitable container and store in the refrigerator until needed.

SLAW DRESSING

Yield: 1½ quarts
Prep time: 15 minutes

Ingredients	Quantity
• Water	1 cup
• Granulated sugar	1 cup
• Rice vinegar	1 cup
• Lemon juice	1 cup
• Fresh ginger, peeled and minced	2 ounces (1 inch)
• Fresh garlic, peeled and minced	2 ounces (1 bulb)
• Jalapeño pepper, stem removed, seeded and chopped	1 small pepper
• Canola oil	1½ cups
• Salt and white pepper mix (p. 211)	2 teaspoons

Step	Procedure
1	Combine the water, sugar, vinegar, lemon juice, ginger, garlic, and jalapeño pepper in a blender or food processor. Blend until smooth.
2	While the machine is running, remove the top and slowly add the oil in a steady stream.
3	Season with the salt and white pepper mix.
4	Transfer the vinaigrette into a suitable container and store in the refrigerator until needed.

Variations: This dressing can be used as a marinade for chicken or pork. To make a cold sauce, combine 1 cup of soy sour cream with ½ cup of slaw dressing.

SPICY TOMATO VINAIGRETTE

Yield: 1 quart
Prep Time: 15 minutes

Sambal oelek contains distilled vinegar (corn) and sulfites (see following box). If there is a concern about these ingredients, you can substitute 1 teaspoon crushed chili flakes for the sambal oelek.

Ingredients	Quantity
• Diced tomatoes, no salt added	2 each, 14.5 ounce cans
• Sambal oelek	2 teaspoons
• Olive oil	½ cup
• Fresh oregano, stems removed	4 tablespoon
• Fresh parsley, stems removed	2 tablespoons
• Balsamic vinegar	2 tablespoons
• Salt and white pepper mix (p. 211)	½ teaspoon

Step	Procedure
1	Combine the tomatoes, sambal oelek, oil, oregano, parsley, and balsamic vinegar in a blender; puree until smooth.
2	Add the salt and white pepper mix and blend for 10 seconds to combine the ingredients.
3	Transfer the vinaigrette into a suitable container and store in the refrigerator until needed.

Safety tip: Read red chili flakes ingredient list. I have found some cheaper brands that state they may contain wheat, soy, and milk allergens.
Variations: You can substitute 28 ounces of roasted tomatoes for the fresh tomatoes to make roasted tomato vinaigrette.

SOUPS AND STEWS

Soups and stews are comfort foods that are popular guest items. I don't know many people that do not like a good cup of soup with a salad. I am one of them. You may have the option to make your own soups but many restaurateurs have premade soups. I prefer to make my soups from scratch because I can control what ingredients are added and they can be prepared in one pot, thus reducing the chance of cross-contact. If you do make your own soups, I have two concerns worth mentioning:

1. If you make two different soups from scratch, use separate utensils to stir each soup and keep the utensils separate from other kitchen tools while in use. This will avoid unwanted food allergens from getting into the soup.
2. Use separate serving ladles to serve the soup. Place the soup with more food allergens in front of the soup with fewer food allergens. During service, someone may inadvertently drip one soup into the other, thus causing the soup to contain unwanted and unknown food allergens.

WHAT ARE SULFITES?

According to the Canadian government, sulfites are one of the nine most common food additives that cause severe adverse reactions. Sulfites are substances that naturally occur in food and the human body. They are also a regulated food additive used as a preservative to maintain food color and prolong shelf life, prevent the growth of microorganisms, and to maintain the potency of certain medications. Sulfites are used to bleach food starches (e.g., potato) and are also used in the production of some food packaging materials (e.g., cellophane).

MANUFACTURED SOUPS

Today more and more restaurants, especially chain restaurants, are serving premade soups to help maintain product quality and consistency. There are advantages and disadvantages to using premade soups.

Advantages

- Many premade soups come frozen in 3-, 5-, or 8-pound bags. These soups can be heated directly in the bag, cut open when hot, and poured directly into a serving pan. This heating procedure reduces the chance of unwanted food allergens being introduced into the soup during heating.
- Premade soups reduce the chance of a cook changing the recipe at the last minute if a certain ingredient was not available.

Disadvantage

- Premade soups contain multiple ingredients that may be unfamiliar to kitchen personnel. Reviewing the ingredient statement may reveal the top eight food allergens listed but there are other ingredients in the soup a person may be allergic to. Always have a copy of the most current package label, even if you have to cut it off the box. This it best way to provide your guest with current ingredient information.

Cream of Broccoli Soup

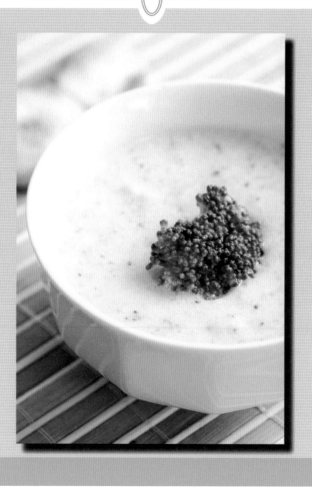

CREAM OF BROCCOLI SOUP

Yield: 2 quarts
Prep time: 20 minutes
Cook time: 20 minutes
Food allergen: Soy

This is a beautiful tasting soup. This soup could actually be referred to as a bisque. If you want a thicker soup replace the water with the All-Purpose (Gravy) Sauce (p. 221).

Ingredients	Quantity
• Garlic oil (p. 208)	2 tablespoons
• Minced garlic	2 teaspoons
• Ginger root, peeled and minced	2 teaspoons
• Yellow onions, small diced	4 ounces
• Water	1 quart
• HACO-Swiss Cuisine Santé Vegetable Stock base	1 ounce
• Soy Béchamel (p. 223)	1 quart
• Broccoli, blanched and chopped	8 ounces
• Fresh parsley, stems removed and chopped	2 tablespoons
• Ground nutmeg	¼ teaspoon
• Salt and white pepper mix (p. 211)	1 teaspoon

Step	Procedure
1	Heat the oil in a stainless steel saucepan over high heat. Add the garlic, ginger, and onions; cook until soft, about 2 minutes, stirring occasionally so the vegetables do not burn.

continued

CREAM OF BROCCOLI SOUP (CONTINUED)

Step	Procedure
2	Add the water and vegetable stock base; bring to a boil, whisking to incorporate the base with the water. Reduce to a simmer; cook for 5 minutes.
3	Add the béchamel sauce; bring to a simmer, cook for 5 minutes, stirring occasionally.
4	Add the broccoli; cook for 5 minutes.
5	Using a hand blender, blend the soup ingredients until it reaches the desired consistency.
5	Add the parsley, nutmeg, and salt and white pepper mix; stir to combine.
6	Garnish with broccoli florets.

Preparation tip: When cooking with soy milk, do not use aluminum-based pans. This will turn the soymilk gray.

ROASTED CHICKEN, KASHA, AND SPINACH SOUP

Yield: 2 quarts
Prep time: 20 minutes if roasted chicken is available, 50 minutes if you have to roast the chicken first and allow it to cool before shredding.
Cook time: 35 minutes

This soup is so light and refreshing that it can be served year round. Kasha is a roasted buckwheat groat that has a nutty flavor.

Ingredients	Quantity
• Olive oil blend	2 tablespoons
• Fresh garlic, minced	1 tablespoons
• Celery, small diced	2 ounces
• Yellow or sweet onion, small diced	4 ounces
• Red bell pepper, ribs removed, small diced	2 ounces
• Jalapeño peppers, seeded and minced	2 tablespoons
• Chicken stock	2½ quarts
• Kasha (cracked granulation)	½ cup
• Roasted chicken, shredded	8 ounces
• Spinach or romaine lettuce, shredded	3 ounces
• Chopped cilantro leaves	2 tablespoons
• Kosher salt	1 tablespoon
• Lemon juice	1 tablespoon

Step	Procedure
1	Heat the oil in a 1-gallon saucepot over medium heat for 30 seconds or until it starts to flow easily in the pot.
2	Add the garlic, celery, onions, and peppers; cook and stir occasionally for 3 minutes.

continued

ROASTED CHICKEN, KASHA, AND SPINACH SOUP
(CONTINUED)

Step	Procedure
3	Add the chicken stock; bring to a boil, then reduce to a simmer.
4	Stir in the kasha and continue to simmer; stirring occasionally for 10 minutes.
5	Stir in the chicken, spinach, cilantro, salt, and lemon juice. Simmer for 5 minutes to heat the chicken, wilt the greens, and combine the flavors.
6	Remove from the heat and serve immediately or hold for service.

Safety tip: Some brands of kasha are not gluten-free because of cross-contact during growing, harvesting, transportation, and processing. Birkett Mills is a certified gluten-free manufacturer that produces whole grain buckwheat products.
Product tip: Quinoa or rice can be used in place of the kasha. Adjust cooking times based on the grain used.

MARY'S MINESTRONE

Yield: 2 quarts
Prep time: 20 minutes
Cook time: 20 minutes

Mary made this soup for me while we were dating. It is so good when I came across this recipe it brought back memories of all the great meals we have had together, so I had to include it in this book. Everyone loves a great soup.

continued

MARY'S MINESTRONE (CONTINUED)

Ingredients	Quantity
• Herb oil (p. 209)	2 tablespoons
• Diced yellow onions	8 ounces
• Diced celery	4 ounces
• Diced carrots	4 ounces
• Diced green bell peppers	4 ounces
• Head cabbage, shredded	4 ounces
• Garlic cloves, minced	2 each
• Canned diced tomatoes	1 each, 15 ounce can
• Chicken stock	2 quarts
• Canned garbanzo beans, drained and rinsed	2 ounces
• Canned black-eyed peas, drained and rinsed	3 ounces
• Tinkyada Brown Rice Elbow Pasta, cooked	4 ounces
• Fresh thyme, stems removed, chopped	1 teaspoon
• Salt and white pepper mix (p. 211)	1 teaspoon

Step	Procedure
1	Heat the oil in a 1-gallon saucepan over medium-high heat.
2	Add the onions, celery, carrots, peppers, cabbage, and garlic; cook for 3 minutes, stirring often.
3	Add the tomatoes and stock; bring to a boil.
4	Reduce the soup to a simmer; cook for 15 minutes or until the vegetables are tender.
5	Add the garbanzo beans, black-eyed peas, pasta and thyme. Simmer the soup for 5 minutes.
6	Season to taste with the salt and white pepper mix.

PORK, PEAS, & PASTA STEW

Yield: 2 quarts (1 cup per serving)
Prep time: 35 minutes
Cook time: 45–55 minutes

If you do not have demi-glace, HACO-Swiss Cuisine Santé demi-glace powder is a meatless, allergen-free product.

Ingredients	Quantity
• Herb oil (p. 209)	2 tablespoons
• Pork stew meat, trimmed and cut in 1-inch cubes, season with salt and white pepper mix	1 pound
• Canola oil	2 tablespoons
• Red wine	1/3 cup
• Yellow onion, diced	4 ounces (1/2 cup)
• Canned, diced tomatoes	15 ounces (1½ cups)
• Demi-glace	2 cups
• Bay leaf	1 each
• Frozen peas	5 ounces (1 cup)
• Assorted mushrooms, sliced	6 ounces (2 cups)
• Salt and white pepper mix (p. 211)	1 teaspoon
• Fresh rosemary, chopped	1 teaspoon
• Tinkyada Elbow Brown Rice Pasta, cooked	4 cups
• Parsley, chopped	3 tablespoons

Step	Procedure
1	Heat the oil in a 4-quart saucepan over medium-high heat for 30 seconds, stirring constantly.
2	Add the onions; cook for 1 minute, stirring occasionally.

continued

PORK, PEAS, & PASTA STEW (CONTINUED)

Step	Procedure
3	Add the canola oil and pork; cook for 3–5 minutes, turning often to brown the meat.
4	Add the red wine to deglaze the pan. Stir to remove the browned particles on the bottom of the pan. Reduce the liquid by half.
5	Add the tomatoes and demi-glace; bring to a boil.
6	Add the bay leaf, peas, and mushrooms; reduce to a low simmer, cover and cook for 45 minutes or until the meat is tender and the sauce is slightly thick.
7	Remove the lid and add the rosemary and salt and white pepper mix. Simmer for 5 minutes.
8	Portion ½ cup of pasta into a serving bowl and cover with 1 cup of stew. Garnish with chopped parsley.

TRADITIONAL BEEF STEW

Yield: 2 quarts or eight 8-ounce servings
Prep time: 25 minutes
Cook time: 25 minutes

Beef stew is one of the comfort foods that many people crave, especially during the winter months. Unfortunately traditional stews contain gluten and wheat from flour in the roux and other allergens may be present if beef base is used instead of stock made from scratch. Swiss Chalet Fine Foods distributes HACO-Swiss, Cuisine Santé gluten and allergen-free bases for soups, sauces, and stocks that are a tasty, safe, and an economical way to prepare allergen-free foods. I have incorporated its beef-flavored stock and demi-glace brown sauce in this recipe. To replace flour, substitute Expandex®, a modified tapioca starch that has unique binding properties. If you cannot get Expandex®, tapioca flour is a good substitute.

Ingredients	Quantity
• Canola oil	4 tablespoons
• Fresh garlic cloves, minced	1 ounce
• Sweet onions, chopped	8 ounces
• Celery stalks, medium dice	4 ounces
• Carrots, peeled, stew cut	4 ounces
• Stew meat, trimmed, large dice	20 ounces
• Expandex (modified tapioca starch)	½ ounce (1 tablespoon)
• Beef stock, or in place of beef stock, 1 ounce of Cuisine Santé beef-flavored stock added to 1 quart of water	1 quart
• Demi-glace, or in place of demi-glace, 1 ounce Cuisine Santé Demi Glace Brown Sauce added to 2 cups of water	2 cups
• Tomato paste	3 ounces
• Miniature red potatoes	10 ounces
• Dried thyme	½ teaspoon

continued

TRADITIONAL BEEF STEW (CONTINUED)

Ingredients	Quantity
• Bay leaves	2 each
• Salt and white pepper mix (p. 211)	½ teaspoon

Step	Procedure
1	Heat 2 tablespoons of canola oil in a 1-gallon saucepan over medium-high heat. Add the onions, celery, and carrots; sauté for 5 minutes, stirring occasionally to prevent the vegetables from burning.
2	Add the garlic: cook for 1 minute, stirring often.
3	Toss the beef cubes with the Expandex® or tapioca flour. Add the remaining 2 tablespoons of canola oil to the pan and add the beef cubes.
4	Lightly brown the beef by stirring the pieces in the pan with the vegetables, 1–2 minutes.
5	Add the stock, demi-glace, and tomato paste, stirring well to incorporate all of the ingredients. Bring to a boil; cook for 1 minute.
6	Stir in the potatoes, dried thyme, bay leaves; reduce the heat to medium; cover and cook for 15 minutes or until the potatoes are tender.
7	Remove the stew from the heat; stir in the salt and white pepper mix.

Safety tip: Make sure all garnishes have been prepared safely. Do not chop herbs with knives that were not properly washed and sanitized, or use cutting boards that were used to cut other ready-to-eat foods such as bread or sandwiches.

Service tip: Remove the bay leaves before serving. The stew can be garnished with freshly chopped parsley or thyme to add additional flavor and color.

SIDE DISHES

When it comes to cooking and serving people with food allergies, I consider the side dish more important than the protein item on the plate. It is easier to prepare a plain chicken breast safely than a side dish. Many side dishes have multiple ingredients and steps of preparation. An incident of cross-contact may occur with the improper use of a utensil or an addition of a whimsical cook. Having a variety of side dishes that have minimal ingredients, simple cooking techniques, and are familiar to the guest will provide you options to create a magical dining experience for them.

CLASSIC MASHED POTATOES

Yield: 6 servings
Prep time: 5 minutes
Cook time: 12 minutes

Classic mashed potatoes contain butter, milk or heavy cream, and are rich and creamy. This version does not contain the top food allergens, and is lighter and healthier with a nice garlic flavor.

Ingredients	Quantity
• Peeled russet potatoes, large dice	1½ pounds
• Earth Balance Natural Buttery Spread, Soy-Free	2 tablespoons (1 ounce)
• Minced garlic	1 teaspoon
• Chicken stock	½ cup
• Salt and white pepper mix (p. 211)	¼ teaspoon

continued

CLASSIC MASHED POTATOES (CONTINUED)

Step	Procedure
1	Place the cubed potatoes in a medium saucepan with cold water.
2	Bring to a boil; cook for 10–12 minutes or until the potatoes are tender but not mushy. At 8 minutes, test some of the potatoes by piercing them with a fork or knife. If the knife goes through the potato easily, they are done. Strain and set aside the potatoes.
3	Place the pan back on the stove and add the buttery spread; melt.
4	Add the garlic; cook for 30 seconds.
5	Add the stock: simmer for 1 minute.
6	Return the potatoes back to the pan; turn off the heat and mash the potatoes to the desired texture.
7	Season with salt and white pepper mix.

Safety tip: If your menu currently features mashed potatoes, prepare a separate batch using this recipe and keep it in a separate hotbox or portable steam table along with plain roasted turkey, All Purpose (Gravy) Sauce (p. 221), and Carrot and Onion Sauté (p. 282). Now you will have an allergen-free meal to offer your guests.

Variation: To make this a vegan dish, substitute the chicken stock with vegetable stock.

ROASTED RED POTATOES

Yield:	2 pounds
Prep time:	10 minutes
Cook time:	22 minutes
Convection oven temperature:	425°F, high fan

This is one of the best side items for your food allergic guest and can be part of your regular menu. It holds well and can be cooked in small or large batches in a short period of time and reheated if necessary.

Ingredients	Quantity
• Red potatoes, preferably small or C's, washed and quartered	2 pounds
• Herb oil (p. 209)	¼ cup

Step	Procedure
1	Wash and cut the potatoes; place in cold water and store in the refrigerator until needed.
2	Drain the potatoes and remove as much water as possible.
3	Toss the potatoes with the herb oil in a mixing bowl; place on a sheet pan lined with parchment paper and allow space between each potato for even cooking and browning.
4	Roast in the oven for 22 minutes.
5	Transfer the potatoes into a hotel pan and place in a food warmer or on the service line.

Safety tip: To use the potatoes later, chill appropriately. Place 4 ounces of potatoes into parchment paper or aluminum foil along with appropriate meat and vegetable. When you have an order, place in a hot oven, 400°F or higher for 10 minutes to reheat. Serve in the foil or transfer to a plate designated for the food allergic guest.

SWEET POTATO MASH

Yield: 6 servings
Prep time: 10 minutes
Cook time: 25 minutes
Food allergen: Soy

Sweet potatoes are large edible tubers that belong to the morning-glory family and are native to the American tropics. There are many varieties but the two widely grown crops are a pale sweet potato and the darker-skinned variety Americans call "yams." The sweet potato and the yam are actually not related and come from different plants all together. Whereas sweet potatoes are higher in vitamin A and C, yams have a higher sugar and moisture content and taste sweeter when cooked.

Ingredients	Quantity
• Sweet potatoes, peeled and cut into chunks	2 pounds
• Kosher salt	½ teaspoon
• Earth Balance, Natural Buttery Spread, Soy-Free	1 tablespoon
• Soy sour cream	3 ounces
• Agave nectar	2 ounces
• Salt and white pepper mix (p. 211)	To taste

Step	Procedure
1	Prepare the potatoes as directed and place in a 2-quart saucepan with salted cold water. Bring to a boil. Simmer 15–20 minutes, until done. Drain and return potatoes to the pan.
2	Add the Earth Balance, soy sour cream, agave nectar; mash the ingredients together with a potato masher until smooth and creamy.
3	Season to taste with salt and white pepper mix.

Variations: To make this dish soy-free, replace the soy sour cream with equal parts Earth Balance, Soy-Free Natural Buttery Spread.

CARROT AND ONION SAUTÉ

Yield: 4 each, 3-ounce servings
Prep time: 5 minutes
Cook time: 8 minutes

Ingredients	Quantity
• Herb oil (p. 209)	1 tablespoon
• Earth Balance, Natural Buttery Spread, Soy-Free	1 tablespoon
• Fresh garlic, minced	1 teaspoon
• Leeks, white parts only, cut in half and thinly sliced	4 ounces
• Sweet onions, peeled, cut in quarters and thinly sliced	4 ounces
• Carrots, peeled and cut into thin Rondelles	5 ounces
• Salt and white pepper mix (p. 211)	To taste

Step	Procedure
1	Heat the oil and Earth Balance over medium heat in a sauté pan until the Earth Balance is melted.
2	Add the garlic, leeks, onions, and carrots; cook for 3–5 minutes, stirring often, until the vegetables are tender.
3	Season to taste with salt and white pepper mix.

Preparation tip: This recipe can be used as a vegetable base for any en papillote dish you create.

CINNAMON-SUGAR CARROTS

Yield: 4 each, 4-ounce servings
Prep time: 5 minutes
Cook time: 45 minutes
Oven temperature: 425°F

This is one of my favorite vegetable recipes. It is easy to make, holds and reheats well, and the leftovers can be used for soups or sauces.

Ingredients	Quantity
• Carrots, peeled and cut into oblique-cut	1 pound
• Canola oil	1 tablespoon
• Granulated sugar	1 teaspoon
• Ground cinnamon	1/8 teaspoon
• Kosher salt	Dash

Step	Procedure
1	Combine the carrots, oil, sugar, cinnamon, and salt in a mixing bowl; toss to mix ingredients. Wrap the carrots in 2 layers of aluminum foil and seal tightly.
2	Bake in a 425°F oven for 30 to 40 minutes or until the carrots are tender. Pierce a large piece with a sanitary fork. If it is hard to pierce the carrot, continue to cook for 5 minutes at a time.
3	When the carrots are cooked, remove from the oven, and keep warm until needed.

Safety tip: Baking foods wrapped in aluminum foil is a safe way to cook and reheat food. The foil traps the flavors, retains moisture, and keeps the food from coming in contact with potential food allergens.

Preparation tip: The carrots can also be cooled down in the foil and reheated the next day if needed. The unused carrots can be used the next day for a sauce, soup, or a quick vegetable sauté.

JULIENNE VEGETABLES FOR EN PAPILLOTE

Yield: 1 pound
Prep time: 10 minutes
Cook time: 5–7 minutes

Ingredients	Quantity
• Herb oil (p. 209)	4 tablespoons
• Julienne carrots	4 ounces
• Julienne parsnips	4 ounces
• Julienne leeks, white part only	4 ounces
• Sliced button mushrooms	4 ounces
• Salt and pepper mix (p. 211)	1/8 teaspoon

Step	Procedure
1	Heat the oil in a nonstick sauté pan until hot.
2	Add the mushrooms; cook for 1 minute, stirring occasionally.
3	Add the julienne vegetables and salt; cook for 2–3 minutes or until the vegetables are tender, not soft.
4	Set the vegetables aside to cool.
5	Portion 2 ounces of vegetables into the bottom half of a 12-inch by 24-inch sheet of parchment paper and add the desired meat and starch. Wrap in parchment or foil.
6	Bake to order.

Variations: Other root vegetables and mushrooms can be substituted in this recipe.

MULTIGRAIN RICE PILAF WITH FRESH HERBS

Yield: 3 cups
Prep time: 10 minutes
Cook time: 55 minutes

Rice is naturally gluten-free and is one of the least allergenic foods. Rice is available in short, medium, and long grain varieties. I used Lundberg Wild Blend: A Gourmet Blend of Wild & Whole Grain Brown Rice, which is gluten-free.

Ingredients	Quantity
• Garlic oil (p. 208)	1 tablespoon
• Yellow onions, small diced	2 ounces
• Celery, small diced	1 ounce
• Carrots, small diced	1 ounce
• Whole grain rice	1 cup
• Chicken or vegetable stock	2 cups
• Bay leaf	1 each
• Fresh rosemary, chopped	1 teaspoon
• Fresh basil, chopped	1 tablespoon
• Salt and white pepper mix (p. 211)	¼ teaspoon

Step	Procedure
1	Heat the oil in a medium saucepan over medium heat.
2	Add the onions, celery, and carrots; cook, stirring occasionally for 2 minutes.
3	Add the rice; stir to coat the rice with the oil. This will keep the grains from sticking together while cooking and creates a fluffy pilaf.

continued

MULTIGRAIN RICE PILAF WITH FRESH HERBS
(CONTINUED)

Step	Procedure
4	Add the stock and bay leaf; stir once and bring to a boil. Cover and reduce to a low simmer.
5	Simmer for 50 minutes, checking often to make sure the pilaf is not simmering too rapidly and the liquid is not evaporating before the rice is cooked.
6	The rice is done when all the liquid is absorbed and the rice is not crunchy but al dente (a French term for "firm to the tooth").
7	Remove the bay leaf. Stir in the fresh herbs and salt and white pepper mix; let the pilaf rest for 5 minutes so the flavors can blend.

Safety tip: Read ingredient statements carefully. Many food service ready-to-use rice mixes contain ingredients that contain allergens.

SAFFRON-SCENTED BUCKWHEAT PILAF

Yield: 7 cups
Prep time: 10 minutes
Cook time: 25 minutes

According to the National Buckwheat Institute, buckwheat is gluten-free, lowers cholesterol, fights adult onset diabetes, is the highest in balanced protein of any food in the vegetable kingdom, and is often raised organically. It is versatile and can be prepared in many different, delicious, and nutritious ways. Buckwheat is sold in many forms:

- Whole buckwheat groats are hulled and unroasted.
- Kasha is hulled, roasted. and packaged in whole, coarse, medium. and fine grinds.
- Cream of Buckwheat is 100% pure groats milled to the size of sesame seeds.
- Buckwheat flour, both light and whole, are 100% gluten-free.

Buckwheat should only be purchase from a certified gluten-free manufacturer. Birkett Mills out of New York is certified gluten-free, and its groats and kasha are of the highest quality, great tasting, and nutritious.

Ingredients	Quantity
• Olive oil	4 tablespoons
• Yellow onions, small diced	½ cup
• Fresh garlic, minced	2 cloves
• Vegetable stock	4 cups
• Bay leaves	2 each
• Saffron	1/8 teaspoon
• Whole buckwheat groats	2 cups
• Salt and white pepper mix (p. 211)	½ teaspoon

continued

SAFFRON-SCENTED BUCKWHEAT PILAF
(CONTINUED)

Step	Procedure
1	Heat the oil in a large saucepan over medium heat; cook the onions and garlic until the onions are soft and translucent, about 1–2 minutes.
2	Add the vegetable stock; bring to a boil over high heat. Quickly stir in the buckwheat; reduce to a simmer. Add bay leaves and saffron; reduce to a simmer and cover pan tightly.
3	Simmer 15 minutes or until grains are tender and liquid is absorbed. Add salt and white pepper mix to taste. Let the pilaf rest for 5 minutes; fluff with a fork. Remove the bay leaves.
4	The pilaf can be held up to 2 hours in a hotbox or warmer.

ENTREES

Entrees or the "center of the plate" ingredients should be very simple. Stick to plain chicken breasts, pork tenderloin or loin cuts, and steaks. You can simply season these meats with canola or olive oil, and salt and white pepper mix (p. 211), sear in a pan, finish in the oven (covered) and serve with a nice side dish. Your guests will be ecstatic. Remember to keep it simple to keep the guest safe. The following recipes are simple but have a touch of flavor to make them captivating.

Bacon-Wrapped Pork Medallions, Balsamic Fruit Chutney, Seasonal Vegetables, Multigrain Rice Pilaf

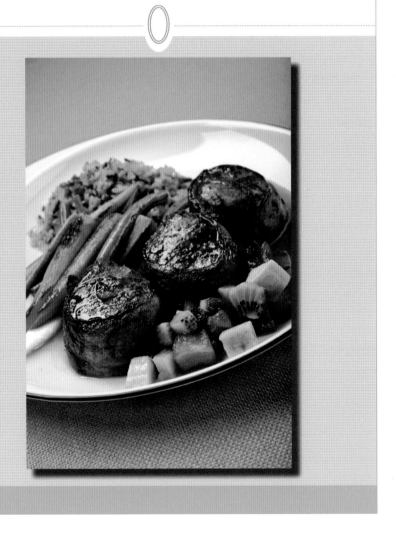

BACON-WRAPPED SPICED PORK MEDALLIONS

Yield: 2 each, 6 ounce servings
Prep time: 15 minutes
Cook time: 12 minutes
Oven temperature: 400°F

Ingredients   Quantity

- Pork tenderloin, cut into 6 each, 2 ounce medallions   12 ounces
- Canola oil   1 tablespoon
- Middle Eastern Spice Mix (p. 210)   2 teaspoons
- Applewood smoked bacon   6 pieces

Step   Procedure

1   Remove the silver skin from the tenderloin. Cut into the
       indicated portion.

2   Rub the pork medallions with canola oil and spice rub;
       coat evenly.

3   Wrap each medallion with 1 piece of bacon. If the bacon does
       not stay attached, secure with a toothpick or skewer.

4   Preheat a nonstick pan over medium-high heat.

5   Sear the bacon where it comes together on the medallion.
       This will keep the bacon from coming unwrapped when
       cooked. Evenly brown the pork on all sides.

6   Sear the top and bottom of each medallion for 30 seconds.

7   Place the medallions on a sheet pan lined with parchment paper
       and bake in the oven for 10 minutes or until the internal
       temperature reaches 145°F. Serve immediately.

Service tip: Serve with Balsamic Fruit Chutney (p. 244), Carrot and Onion Sauté (p. 282),
and Multigrain Rice Pilaf (p. 285).

BREADED TURKEY CUTLET

Yield: 6 servings
Prep time: 25 minutes
Cook time: 20 minutes
Oven temperature: 350°F
Food allergen: Egg

While working at Disney, Mary and I had many opportunities to conduct cooking demonstrations for our guests. One of the opportunities was to participate as guest chefs for the Disney Cruise Line Master Chef Series. On one occasion, Mary and I took a cruise during the Thanksgiving holiday season, so this was a fitting dish to present. This dish is free of many of the top food allergens. I hope you and your guests enjoy it. This can be served with ginger-cranberry chutney, roasted vegetables, and multigrain pilaf.

Ingredients	Quantity
• Chef Joel's All-Purpose Breading Mix (p. 212)	2 cups
• Fresh turkey breast	1 pound
• Salt and white pepper mix (p. 211)	1½ teaspoons
• Whole egg	1 each
• Rice milk	1 cup
• Dry thyme leaves	¼ teaspoon
• Dried oregano leaves	1 teaspoon
• Paprika	¾ teaspoon
• Canola oil	1 cup

Step	Procedure
1	Cut the turkey breast into ¼-inch thick slices; place between 2 sheets of plastic wrap. Pound each piece until you achieve the desired thickness. Season the meat with the salt and white pepper mix.

continued

BREADED TURKEY CUTLET (CONTINUED)

Step	Procedure
2	Follow standard breading procedure used for the Crispy Onion Rings found on p. 304.
	1. Add 1 cup of breading mixture in the first pan.
	2. Whisk together the egg and milk in the second pan.
	3. Mix together the remaining cup of breading mix with the thyme, oregano, and paprika in the third bowl.
3	Dip the product in the breading mixture to coat evenly. Shake off excess.
4	Dip in egg–rice milk mixture to coat completely. Remove. Let excess drain off so the crumb coating will be even.
5	Dip in the final breading mix. Cover with breading and press them gently onto the product. Make sure it is coated completely.
6	Remove. Carefully shake off excess. Fry immediately or hold for service.
7	To fry, preheat a sauté pan over medium-high heat with enough oil to cover the bottom of the pan.
8	Pan-fry the cutlets on both sides until golden brown. Transfer to a sheet pan lined with paper towels. If you are preparing multiple batches, change the oil when the oil starts to get dark with burnt particles.
9	When all of the cutlets are cooked, place on a sheet pan lined with parchment paper; reheat in the oven for 3 minutes and serve.

Lemon Chicken, Cinnamon-Sugar Carrots, & Roasted Potato En Papillote

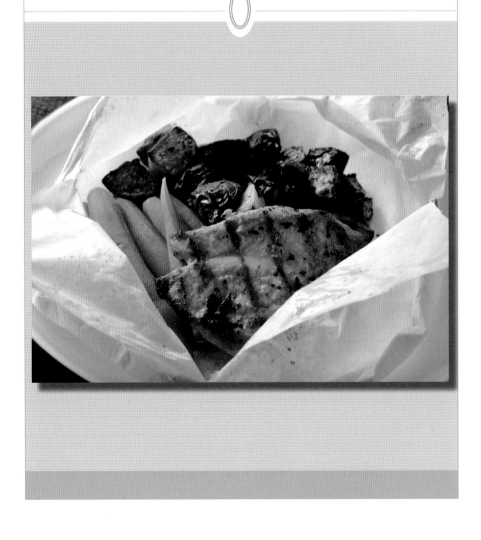

LEMON-HERB CHICKEN BREAST

Yield: 4 servings
Prep time: 10 minutes
Cook Time: 15 minutes

I love the way the herb oil and the fresh citrus blend together to make this a refreshing dish. The longer the chicken marinates the more tender it becomes.

Ingredients	Quantity
• Chicken breasts, trimmed, cut in 4-ounce portions and pounded	1 pound
	2 tablespoons
• Herb oil (p. 209)	1 teaspoon
• Lemon zest	1 tablespoon
• Lemon juice	

Step	Procedure
1	Combine the chicken, herb oil, lemon zest, and juice together in a stainless steel container. Cover and place in the refrigerator to marinate from 4 hours to overnight.
2	Preheat a nonstick grill pan or griddle over medium-high heat. Sear the chicken breast on both sides for 1–2 minutes per side.
3	Arrange the chicken breasts on a sheet pan lined with parchment paper. Cover the chicken and store in the refrigerator until needed.
4	To cook the chicken breasts, place in the oven and cook until the internal temperature reaches 165°F. Serve immediately.

Variations: Orange or limes can be substituted for the lemon along with fresh garlic. The chicken can be served sliced on top of a salad, chopped for a chicken salad, or served on gluten-free bread for a sandwich.

LEMON-HERB CHICKEN EN PAPILLOTE

Yield: 4 servings
Prep time: 10 minutes
Cook time: 20 minutes
Oven temperature: 425°F convection oven, fan speed set on high

En papillote refers to food that is baked inside a wrapping of greased parchment paper. As the food cooks and lets off steam, the parchment paper puffs up into a dome shape. At the table, the paper is cut and peeled back to reveal the food.

Ingredients	Quantity
• Lemon-Herb Chicken Breast (p. 295)	4 pieces
• Roasted Red Potatoes (p. 280)	12 ounces
• Cinnamon-Sugar Carrots (p. 283)	1 pound

Step	Procedure
1	Portion 3 ounces of potatoes, 4 ounces of carrots, and 1 marinated 4-ounce chicken breast onto a 12-inch by 24-inch piece of tin foil or parchment paper.
2	Place the ingredients on one half of the foil or paper, fold over the other half and crimp the edges to enclose the ingredients inside.
3	Place the en papiollote on a sheet pan and bake for 20 minutes.
4	This can be served on a plate in the original package or cut open and slide onto a plate.

Safety tip: Using the en papillote method of food preparation can provide you with unlimited options and meal combinations that can be prepared in your "food allergen safety zone"; heated when needed and served to the food allergic guest safely.
Preparation tip: The ingredients for this entrée can be prepared ahead of time, portioned into parchment paper or tinfoil, and cooked as needed.

WHOLE GRAIN BROWN RICE PASTA PRIMAVERA

Yield: 1 serving
Prep time: 20 minutes
Cook time: 3 minutes

A la primavera is an Italian phrase meaning "spring style" and refers to the use of fresh vegetables (raw or blanched) as a garnish for a variety of dishes. Today's pasta primavera refers to pasta tossed or topped with diced or julienned cooked vegetables. Many dining establishments offer this dish but many versions contain heavy cream or alfredo sauce, which contains milk allergens. I wanted to revisit this classic dish that was prepared with olive oil, fresh garlic, and vegetables, and substituted the wheat-based pasta with Tinkyada Brown Rice Pasta.

Ingredients	Quantity
• Tinkyada Brown Rice Pasta, cooked	4 ounces (1 cup)
• Herb oil (p. 209)	¼ cup
• Chopped fresh garlic	1–2 teaspoons
• Julienne red bell peppers	½ ounce
• Julienne green bell peppers	½ ounce
• Julienne yellow bell peppers	½ ounce
• Blanched, diagonal sliced carrots	½ ounce
• Blanched, sliced green beans	½ ounce
• Quartered seasonal mushrooms	½ ounce
• Vegetable stock (HACO vegetable stock)	¼ cup
• Salt and white pepper mix	¼ teaspoon
• Cheese alternative (optional)	1 ounce
• Fresh parsley, basil, or thyme, chopped for garnish	1 tablespoon

continued

Whole-Grain Brown Rice Pasta Primavera

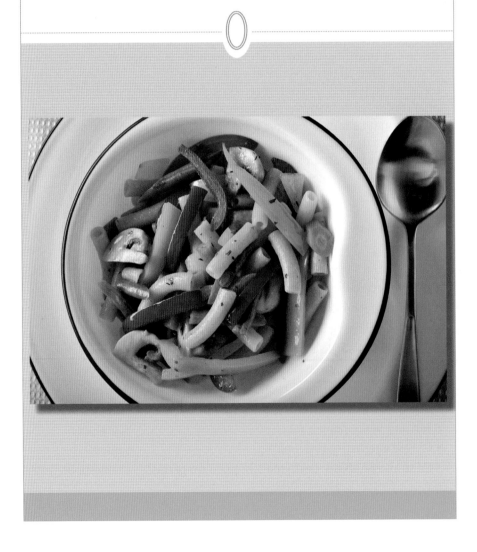

WHOLE GRAIN BROWN RICE PASTA PRIMAVERA
(CONTINUED)

Step	Procedure
1	Cook the pasta as directed on bag (see "Product tip" below). Drain the pasta and run cold water over the pasta to quickly cool it down.
2	Toss the pasta with canola oil to prevent the pasta from sticking together. Portion pasta into 4-ounce portions: bag and refrigerate.
3	Heat the oil in a nonstick sauté pan, over high heat. Add the garlic; cook for 30 seconds.
4	Add the bell peppers, carrots, green beans, and mushrooms; cook, tossing, and stirring often for 2–3 minutes, or until the vegetables are tender.
5	Add the vegetable stock and salt and white pepper mix; cook for 1 minute. Add the pasta and toss to incorporate the ingredients.
6	Transfer to a bowl and garnish with cheese alternative or freshly chopped herbs.

Safety tip: Designate a specific time to prepare your gluten-free and allergen-free foods. Cooking the whole bag of pasta and portioning it will reduce the chance of cross-contact and save you time preparing this dish during service. Always use designated cooking pans and utensils when preparing allergen-free meals.

Product tip: One pound (1 bag) of Tinkyada pasta yields approximately 26 ounces of cooked pasta. I only cook the pasta for 12–14 minutes. When I have cooked it per the package directions, I find the pasta usually is overcooked. It holds better if slightly undercooked. There is a fine line between al dente gluten-free pasta and overcooked gluten-free pasta.

Saffron-Scented Buckwheat Pilaf, Three Bean Salad, Spicy Tomato Vinaigrette

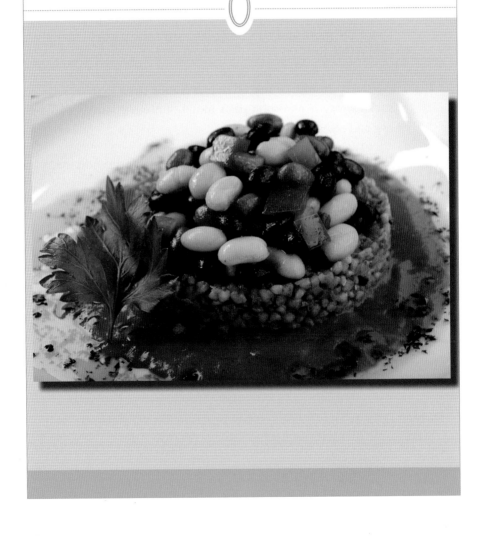

SAFFRON-SCENTED BUCKWHEAT PILAF,
THREE-BEAN SALAD, AND
SPICY TOMATO VINAIGRETTE

Yield: 10 entrée portions

I developed this recipe for an American Culinary Federation presentation I was giving called "Balancing the Plate," which focused on reducing the protein portion size and increasing the whole grains, vegetable, and fruit portions. This dish is completely vegan and has 12 grams of protein and 10 grams of fiber. The first time I made this dish, Mary and I were amazed at the flavors, textures, and how full we felt after eating it.

Ingredients	Quantity
• Saffron Buckwheat Pilaf (p. 287)	1 recipe
• Three-Bean Salad (p. 261)	1 recipe
• Spicy Tomato Vinaigrette (p. 265)	1 recipe
• Herb oil (p. 209)	5 ounces

Step	Procedure
1	Mold the buckwheat pilaf in a ring or greased ramekin. Unmold onto a plate.
2	Pour the spicy tomato vinaigrette around the buckwheat.
3	Drizzle 1 tablespoon of herb oil spicy tomato vinaigrette.
4	Portion the three-bean salad on the buckwheat.
5	Garnish with fresh Italian parsley.

Seared New York Strip, Herb Oil, Crispy Onion Rings, Red Onion Chutney

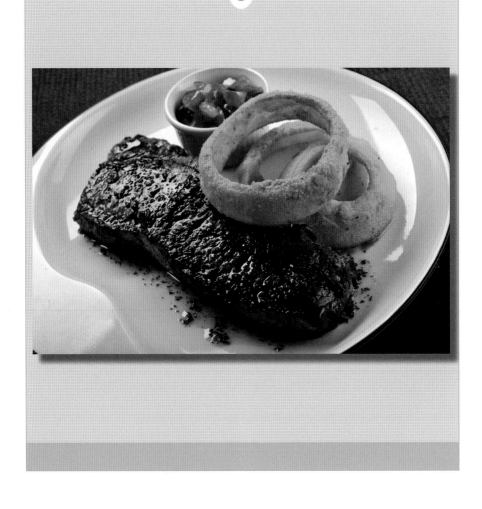

SEARED NEW YORK STRIP STEAK, HERB OIL, CRISPY ONION RINGS, AND RED ONION CHUTNEY

Yield: 1 serving
Prep time: 15 minutes
Cook time: 10 minutes
Oven temperature: 350°F

Mary and I do not eat a lot of red meat but when we looked at the picture of this steak and onion rings, we fell in love with it. Enjoy!

Ingredients	Quantity
• New York strip steak	8 ounces
• Salt and black pepper	To taste
• Herb oil (p. 209)	1 tablespoon
• Crispy Onion Rings (p. 304)	3 each
• Red Onion Chutney (p. 246)	2 ounces

Step	Procedure
1	Season the steak with salt and pepper.
2	Preheat a nonstick griddle or grill pan over high heat.
3	Sear the steak on both sides to add color and flavor to the steak; transfer to a sheet pan lined with parchment paper.
4	Place the steak in the oven and bake until it reaches the desired temperature.
5	Serve the steak on the designated "allergy plate," garnish with the onion rings and serve the chutney on the side.

Service tip: Add Classic Mashed Potatoes (p. 278) and steamed vegetables to make this a complete meal.

CRISPY ONION RINGS

Yield:	12 each, 3 to 4 servings
Prep time:	10 minutes
Cook time:	Depending on cooking method
Oven temperature:	425°F
Fryer temperature:	350°F

These onion rings can be made with different specialty pancake mixes or Chef Joel's All-Purpose Breading Mix (p. 212).

Ingredients	Quantity
• Yellow onions, peeled and cut into ½-inch slices	1 each
• Water, rice milk, or gluten-free beer	¼ cup
• Specialty pancake mix	2 cups
• Garlic powder	½ teaspoon
• Ground red pepper	¼ teaspoon

Step	Procedure
1	Preheat the oven to 450°F or preheat an individual tabletop fryer to 350°F. If you are using the oven, prepare a sheet pan with parchment paper.
2	Set up your "food allergen safety zone" with the standard breading procedure listed below.
3	1. Place the prepared onions in pan 1. 2. Place ½ cup of pancake mix in pan 2. 3. Mix ½ cup of pancake mix with the liquid in pan 3. 4. Mix the remaining pancake mix with the spices and place in pan 4. 5. Have pan 5 ready for the finished product.

continued

CRISPY ONION RINGS (CONTINUED)

Step	Procedure
4	Using disposable food service gloves, take your left hand and place an onion ring in pan 2 and coat the ring thoroughly. Shake off any excess mix before adding it to the next pan.
5	Using the same hand, place the ring into pan 3 and coat the ring thoroughly. Let excess batter drip off before putting it into the next pan.
6	Place the battered ring into pan 4 and using your right hand, coat the ring with the seasoned mix. Transfer the finished product to pan 5. Follow this process for the remaining onion rings.
7	To bake the onion rings, arrange them in a single layer on a sheet pan lined with parchment paper. Bake for 12–18 minutes. Serve immediately.
8	To deep-fry onion rings, place 3 to 4 onion rings at a time into the oil and fry for 3 to 5 minutes, moving them occasionally to prevent sticking. Using designated tongs or strainer, remove the finished rings and place on paper towels to absorb excess oil. Serve immediately.

DESSERTS

The grand finale to any meal is the dessert. A great meal can be ruined if the guest gets a bad dessert or none at all. Since many cakes, cookies, pies, tarts, ice cream, mousse, and custards contain many food allergens, there are not many options for a guest with food allergies except possibly fresh fruit (as long as it is safely prepared). The following recipes offer you options that can be enjoyed by all of your guests, even those without food allergies.

COCONUT RUM TAPIOCA PUDDING

Yield: 1½ quarts
Prep time: 10 minutes
Cook time: 25 minutes
Food allergen: Nuts

Coconuts have been recently added to the nut allergy category.

Ingredients	Quantity
• Small tapioca pearls	1 cup
• Water	2 quarts
• Coconut milk, unsweetened	4 cups
• Brown sugar, light or dark	1 cup (7 ounces)
• Vanilla beans	2 each
• Meyer's dark rum (optional)	4 teaspoons

Step	Procedure
1	Cut the vanilla beans in half, lengthwise. Scrape the seeds; rub the seeds together with the brown sugar. Set aside.
2	Bring the 2 quarts of water to a boil; add the tapioca. Reduce the heat to a low simmer. Cook until the pearls are clear, about 15 minutes, stirring often so the tapioca does not stick to the bottom of the pan. Remove from the heat; strain immediately with a chinois or fine mesh strainer.
3	In another saucepan, add the coconut milk and vanilla bean pods; bring to a simmer. As soon as the coconut milk reaches a low simmer, add the strained tapioca and cook, stirring often for an additional 5 minutes.
4	Add the brown sugar–vanilla bean seeds; simmer for an additional 5 minutes, stirring often.
5	Transfer the tapioca to a stainless steel mixing bowl; chill over an ice bath, stirring occasionally. Add the rum and mix thoroughly. Portion into containers. Chill for 8 hours or overnight before serving.

Lemon Grass Consommé with Seasonal Berries

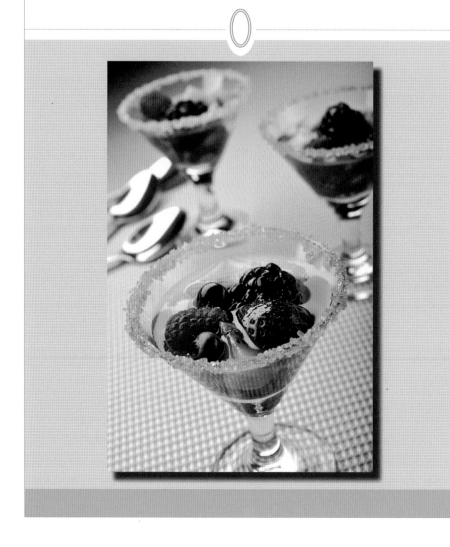

LEMONGRASS CONSOMMÉ WITH FRESH BERRIES

Yield: 2 quarts plus 2/3 cup
Prep time: 25 minutes
Cook time: 20 minutes

Ingredients	Quantity
• Lemongrass stalks	12 each
• Water	8 cups
• Granulated sugar	4 ¼ cups
• Blueberries	½ cup
• Raspberries	1 cup
• Strawberries, quartered	1 cup
• Kiwis, diced	2 each

Step	Procedure
1	Clean, trim, and chop the lemongrass. In a medium saucepan, bring the water and sugar to a boil, dissolving the sugar. Add the chopped lemongrass and reduce the heat. Simmer for 20 minutes.
2	Remove from the heat and cool in an ice bath. Cover and place in cooler overnight.
3	The following day, strain the syrup into a container. Discard the lemongrass. The syrup (consommé) can be stored for 7-10 days in the cooler.
4	Presentation: Sugarcoat the rim of a martini glass by lightly dipping rim of the glass in agave nectar. Then dip in raw sugar. Place an assortment of fresh fruit in the martini glass and fill with lemon grass consommé.

Pumpkin Upside-Down Cake with Caramelized Cranberries

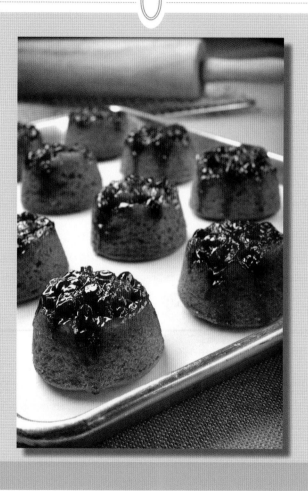

PUMPKIN UPSIDE-DOWN CAKE WITH CARAMELIZED CRANBERRIES

Yield: One 9-inch cake or 10 standard muffins
Prep time: 30 minutes
Cook time: 25 minutes
Food allergen: Eggs

Ingredients	Quantity
For Smear	
• Earth Balance Natural Buttery Spread, Soy-Free	2¼ ounces
• Light brown sugar	2 ounces
For Pumpkin Cake	
• Whole eggs	2 each
• Pumpkin puree	1 cup (8 ounces)
• Light agave nectar	½ cup
• Canola oil	2 tablespoons
• Vanilla extract	1½ teaspoons
• Gluten-free flour blend	2 cups (7 ounces)
• Baking powder	1½ teaspoons
• Baking soda	½ teaspoon
• Ground cinnamon	1½ teaspoons
• Table Salt	¼ teaspoon
• Cranberries, frozen or fresh	1½ cups

Step	Procedure
1	Grease one 9-inch cake pan with Earth Balance Natural Buttery Spread, Soy-Free; line the bottom with parchment paper. Set aside.

continued

PUMPKIN UPSIDE-DOWN CAKE WITH
CARAMELIZED CRANBERRIES (CONTINUED)

Step	Procedure
2	In a saucepan, melt the Earth Balance over medium heat. Add the brown sugar and whisk until smooth and mixture emulsifies. The mixture will look broken and separated before it emulsifies. Pour the brown sugar mixture into the bottom of the prepared pan.
3	When the brown sugar mixture has cooled, arrange the cranberries in a single layer covering the bottom of the pan. Set aside.
4	In a large bowl, whisk together the eggs; add the pumpkin puree, agave nectar, canola oil, and vanilla extract; whisk until smooth. Set aside.
5	In another bowl, sift together the gluten-free flour, baking powder, baking soda, cinnamon, and salt. Whisk to combine.
6	Fold the flour mixture into the pumpkin mixture using a rubber spatula. Carefully spread the batter over the cranberry topping.
7	Bake at 350° F for approximately 35–40 minutes. Let cool for 15 minutes on a wire rack. Place a cake board on top of the cake. Invert the cake with the cake board. Carefully peel off the parchment paper. Let cool completely before serving.

Standard muffins: Place 2 teaspoons of smear into each greased standard muffin cavity. This smear yields enough for 10 muffins. When cool and you are ready to fill with pumpkin batter, place approximately 7 large cranberries in each. Portion a #16 scoop of batter into each cavity. Bake at 375° F for approximately 20–25 minutes. Please note that these baking times are just guidelines.

QUINOA CRÊPES, APPLE BUTTER, AND APPLES

Yield: 4 servings
Prep time: 2 hours
Cook time: 30 minutes

I find that store-bought apple butter works great in this recipe. There are brands that are free from the top eight allergens.

Ingredients	Quantity

For Crêpes

• Gluten-free flour blend	2/3 cup (3 ounces)
• Quinoa flour	½ cup (2 ounces)
• Granulated sugar	8 teaspoons
• Table Salt	¼ teaspoon
• Flax meal	2 tablespoons
• Water	6 tablespoons
• Rice milk	1 cup

For Apple Compote (yields 3 ½ cups)

• Granny Smith apples, peeled, cored, and medium diced	1½ pounds
• Earth Balance Natural Buttery Spread, Soy-Free	1½ tablespoons
• Granulated sugar	1/3 cup plus 1 tablespoon
• Ground cinnamon	¼ teaspoon
• Table Salt	Pinch
• Apple butter	½ cup
• Rice Dream Vanilla Non-Dairy Frozen Dessert	½ quart

continued

Quinoa Crepes, Apple Butter, with Apple Compote

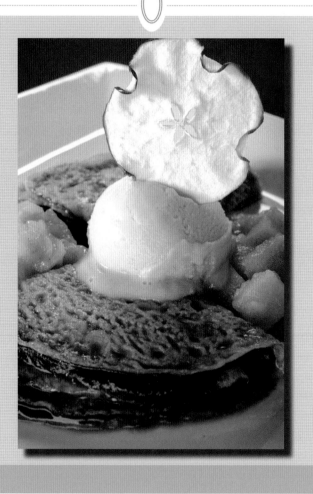

QUINOA CRÊPES, APPLE BUTTER, AND APPLES
(CONTINUED)

Ingredients	Quantity
For Poaching Liquid	
• Water	6 ounces
• Granulated sugar	6 ounces (12 tablespoons)
• Earth Balance Natural Buttery Spread, Soy-Free	6 ounces
• Calvados brandy	6 ounces
• Vanilla extract	1½ teaspoons

Step	Procedure
1	To make the crepes: Combine the gluten-free flour blend, quinoa flour, sugar, and salt. Set aside.
2	Whisk together the flax meal and water. Let this mixture rest for a couple of minutes. Whisk again until mixture is gelatinous. Add the rice milk to the flax mixture and whisk until smooth.
3	Gradually whisk the rice milk mixture into the dry mixture.
4	Let the batter rest in the refrigerator for 2 hours.
5	Preheat a 10-inch nonstick skillet. Using a paper towel, brush the bottom and sides of the skillet very lightly with canola oil.
6	Tilt the pan slightly and begin pouring a scant ¼ cup batter. Continue to pour the batter in a slow, steady stream, rotating your wrist and twirling the pan slowly until the pan is covered with an even layer of batter.
7	Place the cooked crêpe on a plate and repeat the cooking process with the remaining batter, brushing the pan very lightly with canola oil before making each crêpe.

continued

QUINOA CRÊPES, APPLE BUTTER, AND APPLES
(CONTINUED)

Step	Procedure
8	To make the apple compote: Peel, core, and dice the apples.
9	In a saucepan, bring the Earth Balance to a sizzle over high heat. Add the 1½ pounds of diced apples and toss in the Earth Balance. Reduce the heat to medium and cover the pan. Cook, stirring frequently, until the apples are soft but still al dente, about 7–10 minutes.
10	Combine the sugar, cinnamon, and salt. Stir sugar mixture into the apples and increase the heat. Cook, uncovered at a rapid boil for about 3 minutes, until a thick syrup is achieved. Remove from the heat.
11	To make the poaching liquid: Heat the water and sugar for approximately 2 minutes to dissolve the sugar. Add the Earth Balance, Calvados, and vanilla, and simmer for approximately 2 minutes. Keep at a low simmer.
12	To assemble: Spread each crepe with 2 teaspoons of apple butter. Float the crepe, apple butter side up in the hot liquid to reheat the crepe. Do not let the crepe submerge in the liquid. Carefully remove the crepe and fold the crepe in half and in half again. Repeat with the remaining crepes. Arrange 2 quartered crepes on a plate, points touching. Garnish with ¼ cup of apple compote and Rice Dream Vanilla Non-Dairy Frozen Dessert.

Safety tip: To minimize the possibility of any food allergens coming in contact with a specialty frozen dessert, designate a colored-handle portion scoop to use for this task. Have this piece of equipment in your "allergen-free zone" or in the designated storage container along with your other allergen-free tools. You can also prescoop a whole container of the frozen dessert and store them in a sealed container in the freezer. This will make it easy to find and serve with the dessert.

RICE PUDDING WITH AGAVE NECTAR
AND SEASONAL MELON

Yield: 3½ cups
Prep time: 15 minutes
Cook time: 25 minutes
Food allergen: Nuts

Ingredients	Quantity
• Rice milk	2 ¼ cups (18 ounces)
• Coconut milk, unsweetened	2¼ cups (18 ounces)
• Cinnamon stick	1 each, 2 inches
• Arborio rice	¾ cup (5 ounces)
• Light agave nectar	2 ounces
• Table Salt	Pinch
• Cantaloupe	1 small
• Honeydew	1 small

Step	Procedure
1	Bring the rice milk and coconut milk to a boil. Add the Arborio rice and cinnamon stick; simmer for 30–40 minutes on low heat, until the rice is tender, stirring frequently to prevent burning. After 20 minutes of cooking, remove the cinnamon stick.
2	Add the agave nectar and salt to the rice mixture; cook for an additional 5 minutes.
3	Portion 7.5 ounces of rice pudding into each container. Chill. When ready to serve, garnish with fresh cantaloupe and honeydew melon balls.

Rice Pudding with Agave Nectar, Seasonal Melons

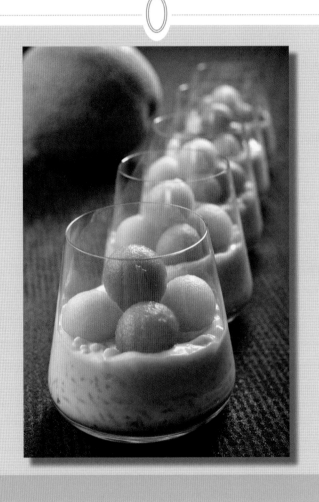

KID DESSERTS

If you really want to make a mother happy, have some allergy-friendly desserts for their kids. I have seen how a simple, packaged cookie or brownie can make a child's face light up and the mother actually cry with tears of joy. I have included two easy desserts that incorporate packaged snacks that can be turned into a fun dessert or be handy for a quick take-away treat.

If your operation has a retail section, these packaged items can be part of your regular offerings and enhance the overall dining experience for these guests.

Chocolate Chip Cookie "Ice Cream" Sandwich

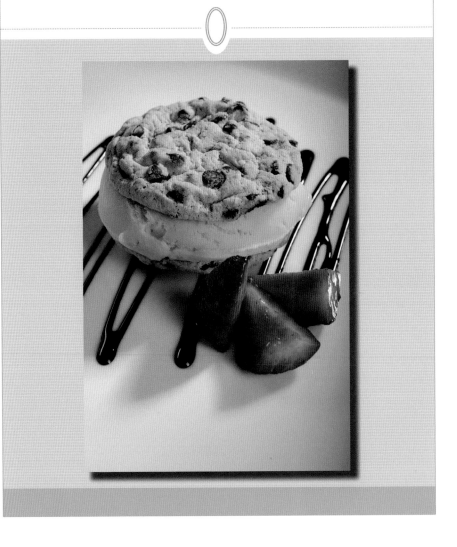

CHOCOLATE CHIP COOKIE "ICE CREAM" SANDWICH

Yield: 1 serving
Prep time: 10 minutes
Food allergens: Wheat, soy

I met Mark Sandler, owner of Divvies, many years ago when he visited me at Disney to introduce his products. He and his wife started this company because their two children have food allergies to the Big 4: milk, egg, peanut, and tree nut. I really like their products because the cookies taste great and are designed to meet these specific allergies.

Ingredients	Quantity
• Divvies® Chocolate chip cookies	2 each
• Rice Dream Vanilla Non-Dairy Frozen Dessert	1 each, 4 ounce scoop
• Fresh strawberries	½ cup
• Granulated sugar	1 tablespoon
• Hershey's Double Chocolate Sundae Syrup	½ ounce

Step	Procedure
1	Drizzle chocolate syrup on plate.
2	Place a scoop of Rice Dream Vanilla Non-Dairy Frozen Dessert between the chocolate chip cookies. Press the cookies together gently.
3	Place the ice cream sandwich on the plate and garnish with sliced strawberries.

Safety tip: Make this dessert ahead of time, individually wrap and freeze until needed. One quart of Rice Dream Non-Dairy Frozen Dessert will yield 8 cookie sandwiches.

Fudge Brownie, "Ice Cream" and Fresh Strawberries

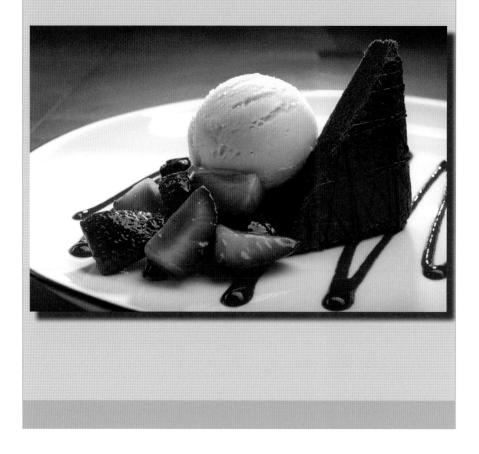

FUDGE BROWNIE, "ICE CREAM,"
AND FRESH BERRIES

Yield: 1 serving
Prep time: 10 minutes
Food allergen: Eggs

Ingredients	Quantity
• French Meadow Bakery Fudge Brownie	1 each
• Rice Dream Vanilla Non-Dairy Frozen Dessert	1 each, 4 ounce scoop
• Raspberry sauce	½ ounce

Step	Procedure
1	Drizzle raspberry sauce on the plate.
2	Cut the brownie in half, diagonally. Arrange the brownie halves on the plate.
3	Serve with a scoop of Rice Dream Vanilla Non-Dairy Frozen Dessert.
4	Garnish with fresh strawberries.

Safety tip: If the guest is unfamiliar with French Meadow Bakery's products, present the guest with the wrapped brownie so he or she can read the ingredient list. There may be times when you can just give the guest the wrapped brownie and the guest will be happy.

GLUTEN-FREE GRANOLA WITH
A POLYNESIAN TWIST

Yield: Makes about 6 cups
Allergen: Nuts

This granola is not only gluten-free, it is free of all the other major allergens, except nuts. You can use any combination of nuts you prefer or happen to have on hand. If nuts are a problem, you can use raw, hulled sunflower or pumpkins seeds instead. This recipe can be easily scaled to serve larger groups.

Ingredients	Quantity
• Gluten-free rolled oats*	2 cups
• Dried unsweetened coconut flakes (not shredded coconut)	1 cup
• Raw cashews, coarsely chopped	½ cup
• Sliced almonds	¼ cup
• Macadamia nuts	¼ cup
• Ground Cinnamon	1 teaspoon
• Sea salt	½ teaspoon
• Honey	1/3 cup
• Canola oil	¼ cup
• Boiling water	¼ cup
• Pure vanilla extract	1 tablespoon
• Chopped dried pineapple	½ cup
• Chopped dried mango	½ cup
• Dried banana chips	½ cup
• Finely chopped candied ginger	¼ cup
• Dried cranberries	¼ cup

continued

GLUTEN-FREE GRANOLA WITH A
POLYNESIAN TWIST (CONTINUED)

Step	Procedure
1	Preheat the oven to 300°F. Line a large (18 inch × 13 inch) baking sheet with parchment paper.
2	In a large bowl, whisk together the oats, coconut, cashews, almonds, macadamia nuts, cinnamon, and salt until well blended.
3	In a small bowl, whisk together the honey, oil, water, and vanilla until blended. Pour evenly over the oat mixture and toss until all ingredients are well moistened. Spread the mixture evenly on the baking sheet.
4	Bake until lightly browned, stirring occasionally, about 20 to 25 minutes. Cool the granola on the baking sheet on a wire rack. When cool; stir in the pineapple, mango, banana chips, ginger, and cranberries. Store, tightly covered, in a dark, dry place for up to 3 days.

Source: Carol Fenster, author of *100 Best Gluten-Free Recipes* (Wiley, 2010).
* Available from BobsRedMill.com; CreamHillEstates.com; GlutenFreeOats.com; GiftsofNature.net; and OnlyOats.ca.

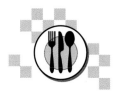

APPENDIX:
SUPPORT ORGANIZATIONS,
BOOKS, SPECIALTY
EQUIPMENT, AND INDEX

SUPPORT ORGANIZATIONS

Autism Society of America
4340 East-West Hwy, Suite 350
Bethesda, Maryland 2081
Phone: 301-657-0881 or 800-3AUTISM (800-328-8476)
Web site: www.autism-society.org

Autism Network for Dietary Intervention (ANDI)
P.O. Box 335
Pennington, NJ 08534-0335
Phone: 609-737-8985
Fax: 609-737-8453
Web site: www.autismndi.com

American Academy of Allergy Asthma & Immunology
Phone: 414-272-6071
E-mail: info@aaaai.org
Web site: www.aaaai.org

American Celiac Disease Alliance (ACDA)
Phone: 730-622-3331
E-mail: info@americanceliac.org
Web site: www.americanceliac.org

The American Diabetes Association
P.O. Box 11454
Alexandria, VA 22312
Phone: 800-DIABETES (800-342-2383)
Web site: http://www.diabetes.org

Anaphylaxis Canada
Phone: 416-785-5666
Web site: www.anaphylaxis.org

The Asthma and Allergy Foundation of America (AAFA)
Phone: 800-727-8462
E-mail: info@aafa.org
Web site: www.aafa.org

Canadian Allergy, Asthma and Immunology Foundation
Phone: 613-730-6272
Web site: www.allergyfoundation.ca

Canadian Celiac Association (CCA)
Phone: 800-363-7296
E-mail: info@celiac.ca
Web site: www.celiac.ca

Canadian Diabetes Association
Phone: 800-226-8464
Web site: www.diabetes.ca

Celiac Disease Foundation (CDF)
Phone: 818-990-2354
E-mail: cdf@celiac.org
Web site: www.celiac.org

Celiac Sprue Association/USA, Inc. (CSA)
Phone: 877-272-4272
E-mail: celiacs@csaceliacs.org
Web site: www.csaceliacs.org

Dietitians of Canada
Phone: 416-596-0857
Web site: www.dietitians.ca

The Food Allergy & Anaphylaxis Network (FAAN)
Phone: 800-929-4040
E-mail: faan@foodallergy.org
Web site: www.foodallergy.org

Gluten Intolerance Group of North America (GIG)
Phone: 253-833-6655
E-mail: info@gluten.net
Web site: www.gluten.net

National Foundation of Celiac Awareness (NFCA)
Phone: 215-325-1306
E-mail: infor@celiaccentral.org
Web site: www.celiaccentral.org

RESOURCE BOOKS

The Complete Guide to Food Allergy and Intolerance, 4th Edition
Authors: Professor Jonathan Brostoff and Linda Gamlin

The Food Intolerance Bible
Authors: Antony J. Haynes and Antoinette Savill

On the Nature of Food Allergy
Author: Paul J. Hannaway, MD

The CalorieKing®: Calorie, Fat, & Carbohydrate Counter, 20th
  Anniversary Edition
Author: Allan Borushek
Web site: www.calorieking.com

Let's Eat Out with Celiac/Coeliac & Food Allergies! 3rd **Edition**
Authors: Kim Koeller and Robert La France
Web site: www.glutenfreepassport.com or www.allergyfreepassport.com

Food Allergies for Dummies
Authors: Robert Wood, MD, and Joe Kraynak

COOKBOOKS AND MAGAZINES

Carol Fenster, PhD, founder and president of Savory Palate, Inc.
8174 So. Holly, #404
Centennial, CO 80122-4004
Phone: 800-741-5418
Web site: www.savorypalate.com

- Gluten-Free 101
- Gluten-Free Quick & Easy
- Cooking Free
- Wheat-Free Recipes & Menus
- 1000 Gluten-Free Recipes
- 100 Best Gluten-Free Recipes

Gluten-Free Baking with The Culinary Institute of America: 150
  Flavorful Recipes from the World's Premier Culinary College
Authors: Richard J. Coppedge Jr., CMB

Gluten-Free Diet: A Comprehensive Resource Guide, **Revised and**
  Expanded Edition
Authors: Shelley Case, BSc, RD
Web site: www.glutenfreediet.ca

MAGAZINES

Allergic Living
Allergies, Asthma, and Gluten-Free
Web site: www.allergicliving.com

Gluten-Free Living
Leading the Way to a Happy, Healthy Gluten-Free Life
Web site: www.glutenfreeliving.com

Living Gluten-Free for Dummies
Author: Danna Korn, founder of the national support group R.O.C.K.
  (Raising Our Celiac Kids)

Living Without
The magazine for people with allergies and food sensitivities
Web site: www.livingwithout.com

SPECIALTY EQUIPMENT— CHEF JOEL'S RECOMMENDATIONS

Allergen Saf-T-Zone™ System Tools

- The Purple Board™, available in three sizes
- Color-coded 10" chefs knife, 12" stainless steel tongs and turner (spatula).

SAN JAMAR
Phone: 262-723-6133
Customer Care: 800-248-9826
E-mail: CustomerCare@sanjamar.com
Web site: www.sanjamar.com

Grill and Griddle Pans

- Cuisinart® GreenGourmet® Hard Anodized 11-inch Square Grill Pan
- Calphalon® Contemporary Nonstick 11-inch Griddle

Cooking Equipment

- All-Clad® Classic Waffle Maker available at Williams-Sonoma
- Black & Decker® Home, Countertop Toaster Ovens; http://www.blackanddeckerappliances.com/c-23-ovens-toasters.aspx
- FryDaddy™ Electric Deep Fryer available at most department stores
- Krups, KJ 7000 High-Performance Deep Fryer available at Williams-Sonoma
- Oster® Digital Food Steamer; http://www.oster.com/ProductDetails.aspx?pid=2002

Special Plate

- Corelle® Contours, Edgy; Customer Care Center, 800-999-3436; http://www.corelle.com/index.asp?pageId=72

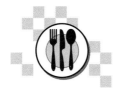

INDEX

Immunoglobulin E (IgE), 4. *See also* IgE antibodies
Incidental additives, ingredient declaration, 30
Incorrect information, 144
Individual packages, 203
Individual pans, *vs.* common cooking equipment, 160
Individually packed items, 176
Inflammation, 14
Inflammatory bowel disease, 78
Ingestion, 18
Ingredient books, 147
Ingredient labeling, 18
  checking with guest, 133–134, 167–168
Ingredient statements, 18, 26, 156
  checking, 133
  obtaining from suppliers, 176
  reviewing for prepared foods, 153
  updating, 110
Inhalation, 17
Inner cities
  hygiene and allergies, 20
  indoor allergens in, 20
Insulin-dependent diabetes, 87
Insulin resistance, 88
Intellectual and developmental disabilities (IDD), 92, 94
Ipad, 133
Iphones, apps for, 133
Ipod Touch, 133
Irritable bowel syndrome (IBS), 78
Itching, 16
  oral, 16

J

Japan, food allergy statistics, 9
JJ's Seafood Bar & Grill, 111
Julienne vegetables, for en papillote, 284
Juvenile-onset diabetes, 87

K

Kapiolani Community College, xviii
Kettle Cuisine, 184

Kinnikinnick Foods, 185
Kitchen equipment, 159
Kitchen management, 143
  4R's for, 164–172
  at-table guest visit, 167–168
  checking preparation procedure, 169
  flow of food, 143–144
  food allergy review with guest, 167–168
  guest communication prior to visit, 164–166
  HACCP plan for food allergen safety, 144–164
  ingredient label checking, 167–168
  kitchen preparation for food allergy requests, 166–167
  referral to chef/manager, 164
  response to guest, 171–172
  taking the order, 168–169
Kitchen staff downsizing, 157
Kitchen tools, 157, 159

L

Labor costs, implications for kitchen management, 143
Lactalbumin, 43, 47, 48
Lactase enzyme pills, 92
Lactic acid, 48
Lacto vegetarians, 96
Lactose, 48
Lactose intolerance, 71, 91
  ethnic distribution, 91
  serving guests with, 92
  symptoms, 92
Las Vegas, improvements in food service awareness, 13
Latex allergy, 157, 158, 166
Lawsuits, protection through labeling, 25
Lead server, 107, 108
Lecithin, 60
Legal consultants, 107, 108, 109
Legal disclaimer, 112
Legumes, 49
Lemon chocolate-chip scones, 235–238